DR. GEORGINA TRACY

THE
ULTIMATE
ALL-IN-ONE GUIDE
TO REVERSE KIDNEY STONE WITH EASY COOKING

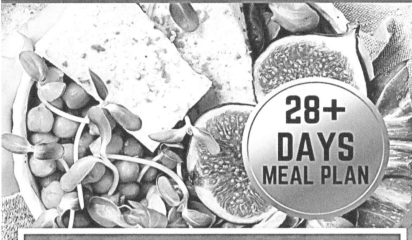

28+ DAYS MEAL PLAN

KIDNEY STONE
DIET
COOKBOOK

KIDNEY STONE

DIET

COOKBOOK

The Ultimate All-In-One Guide to Reverse Kidney Stone with Easy Cooking.

DR. GEORGINA TRACY

Table of Contents

FOREWORD

Hi there!

I'm delighted to welcome you to the KIDNEY STONE DIET COOKBOOK. This cookbook is not just a collection of recipes, but a testament to the power of nutrition and dieting in overcoming kidney stone complications. Let me share with you a brief record of a personal journey of survival and triumph all thanks to nutrition.

Not too long ago, my elder brother found himself in the grip of an excruciating pain that turned out to be a kidney stone. According to him, the pain was unbearable, and he was desperate for a solution. He had phoned me past midnight one day, lamenting on how terrible he felt, and with that, we both decided he'd be visiting the hospital first thing once the sun was up.

Luckily, his case was diagnosed early. After undergoing some level of medical treatment, he realized that he needed to take charge of his health and make some lifestyle changes, including his diet.

With a determination to fight back, he delved into the world of nutrition, and with my help, researched extensively on how to manage kidney stones through diet. He learned that certain foods can aggravate kidney stones, while others can help prevent and reverse their formation. Using his records, together, we carefully crafted his meals, choosing ingredients that were kidney stone-friendly, and experimenting with flavors and textures to make my meals enjoyable and satisfying.

The results were nothing short of miraculous! Not only did he successfully manage and reverse his kidney stones, but he also experienced an overall improvement in my kidney health. It was a wake-up call for Dylan, my brother – he realized the power of food in supporting our health and well-being, and we were inspired to share this knowledge with others who may be facing similar challenges.

And that's how the KIDNEY STONE DIET COOKBOOK came to be. In this cookbook, you'll find a treasure trove of delicious recipes that are specifically designed to support kidney health. From scrumptious breakfasts to mouthwatering dinners, from comforting soups to tempting desserts, every recipe is carefully crafted with the right balance of nutrients and flavors to help you manage kidney stones and promote optimal kidney health.

But this cookbook is not just about recipes. It's also about empowering you with knowledge. You'll learn about the science behind kidney stones and how different foods can impact kidney health. You'll discover the key nutrients that are beneficial for kidney health, and how to incorporate them into your diet. You'll also find practical tips on how to grocery shop, meal plan, and cook with kidney health in mind.

I know firsthand that managing or dieting for kidney stones reversal can be challenging, but it's also incredibly rewarding. Through my brother's journey, I've come to appreciate the joy of cooking and the immense impact that food can have on our health even more. I've discovered new ingredients, flavors, and culinary techniques that have enriched my life in so many ways. Cooking has become not just a necessity but also a creative outlet and a source of joy for me, and I hope that this cookbook inspires you to experience the same.

I want to express my heartfelt gratitude to everyone who has supported me on this journey, from Dylan, my family and friends, to the chefs and co-medical professionals who have guided me along the way. Your unwavering support has been my driving force, and I'm thrilled to share my knowledge and experience with you in this cookbook.

So, let's embark on this culinary adventure together! Let's savor the delicious recipes, nourish our bodies, and celebrate the power of nutrition and dieting in managing kidney stones. Here's to a healthier, happier you!

Bon appétit,

Dr. Georgina Tracy.

CHAPTER 1: INTRODUCTION TO KIDNEY STONES AND DIET

What are kidney stones?

Kidney stones, also known as renal calculi, are hard deposits that form in the kidneys. They are composed of minerals and salts, such as calcium, oxalate, uric acid, cystine, and struvite, which crystallize and accumulate in the urinary tract. Kidney stones can vary in size from a grain of sand to a golf ball and can cause severe pain and discomfort as they pass through the urinary tract.

Kidney stones are a common medical condition, affecting approximately 1 in 10 people worldwide. They can form due to various factors, including diet, dehydration, genetics, medical conditions, medications, lifestyle, and other risk factors. The exact cause of kidney stone formation is often multifactorial and can involve a combination of these factors.

Causes and risk factors

Kidney stones can form due to various causes and risk factors, which can increase the likelihood of their formation. These causes and risk factors include:

Diet: Diet plays a significant role in kidney stone formation. Consuming excessive amounts of certain foods high in oxalate, such as spinach, beets, nuts, chocolate, and certain beverages like tea and coffee, can increase the risk of developing calcium oxalate stones, which are the most common type of kidney stones. Diets high in salt, sugar, and animal protein, and low in fruits and vegetables, can also increase the risk of kidney stone formation.

Dehydration: Inadequate fluid intake can lead to dehydration, which can result in concentrated urine. Concentrated urine can promote the crystallization of minerals and salts, leading to the formation of kidney stones. Hot climates, excessive sweating, certain medical conditions (such as diabetes and cystic fibrosis), and certain medications (such as diuretics) can increase the risk of dehydration and kidney stone formation.

Genetics: Family history of kidney stones can increase the risk of developing kidney stones. Research has identified certain genes that may be associated with kidney stone formation, suggesting a genetic predisposition to stone formation.

Medical conditions: Certain medical conditions can increase the risk of kidney stone formation. Conditions such as hyperparathyroidism, cystinuria (a rare genetic disorder that causes excessive cystine in the urine), renal tubular acidosis (a condition that affects the body's ability to regulate acid-base balance), and urinary tract infections can increase the risk of kidney stone formation.

Medications: Some medications can increase the risk of kidney stone formation in susceptible individuals. For example, diuretics (water pills) can increase urine concentration, which can lead to stone formation. Calcium-containing antacids, when taken in excess, can increase the risk of calcium-based kidney stones. Certain antibiotics, such as sulfonamides and fluoroquinolones, can also increase the risk of kidney stone formation.

Lifestyle factors: Sedentary behavior and obesity have been associated with an increased risk of kidney stone formation. Lack of physical activity can lead to decreased urine production and increased urinary stasis, which can promote stone formation. Obesity can increase urinary calcium excretion and decrease urine citrate levels, which can contribute to stone formation.

Urinary tract abnormalities: Structural abnormalities in the urinary tract, such as congenital abnormalities, kidney cysts, or previous urinary tract surgeries, can increase the risk of kidney stone formation. These abnormalities can disrupt normal urine flow, promote urinary stasis, and provide sites for stone formation.

Other factors: Other factors that may contribute to kidney stone formation include history of gastric bypass surgery, prolonged immobilization (such as bedrest or long-haul flights), and certain medical conditions that affect the absorption or metabolism of minerals, such as Crohn's disease, inflammatory bowel disease, and hyperoxaluria (a condition characterized by excessive oxalate in the urine).

It's important to note that not everyone with these risk factors will develop kidney stones, and some individuals without these risk factors may still develop kidney stones. The formation of kidney stones is often multifactorial, and a combination of risk factors can increase the likelihood of their development.

Understanding the causes and risk factors for kidney stones is essential in preventing their formation and recurrence. Lifestyle modifications, dietary changes, staying hydrated, and managing underlying medical conditions can all play a role in reducing the risk of kidney stone formation.

Role of diet in kidney stone prevention

The role of diet in kidney stone prevention is crucial, as certain dietary habits can either contribute to the formation of kidney stones or help prevent their occurrence. Dietary modifications can be an effective strategy to reduce the risk of kidney stone formation or recurrence, and it is often recommended as part of the overall management plan for individuals with a history of kidney stones or who are at increased risk of developing them.

Here, we will discuss in detail the different aspects of diet that play a role in kidney stone prevention:

Fluid intake: Staying hydrated is essential for kidney stone prevention. Drinking an adequate amount of fluids, especially water, helps to increase urine volume, dilute urine, and promote urine flow, which can help flush out potential stone-forming substances from the kidneys and urinary tract.

The goal is to drink enough fluids to produce at least 2 to 2.5 liters (about 8 to 10 cups) of urine per day. In hot climates, during physical activity, or when at increased risk of dehydration, it is important to increase fluid intake accordingly.

However, excessive fluid intake should also be avoided, as it can lead to overhydration and other health issues.

Calcium intake: Contrary to popular belief, calcium is not directly responsible for the formation of calcium-based kidney stones. In fact, adequate dietary calcium intake may actually help reduce the risk of kidney stone formation.

Calcium binds with oxalate in the intestine, preventing its absorption and reducing the amount of oxalate that can be excreted in the urine, thus lowering the risk of calcium oxalate stone formation. Good dietary sources of calcium include dairy products, fortified foods, leafy green vegetables, and calcium supplements as recommended by a healthcare professional.

Oxalate intake: Oxalate is a naturally occurring substance found in many plant-based foods, and high levels of oxalate in urine can contribute to the formation of calcium oxalate stones, which are the most common type of kidney stones. Therefore, it is important to limit the intake of foods high in oxalate, such as spinach, beets, nuts, chocolate, and certain beverages like tea and coffee.

However, it is important to note that oxalate from food is not the only factor that influences oxalate levels in urine, as oxalate is also produced by the body and can be influenced by other factors like gut health and genetics.

Sodium intake: High dietary sodium (salt) intake can increase the risk of kidney stone formation, as it can lead to increased urinary calcium excretion and decreased urine citrate levels, both of which can contribute to stone formation. Therefore, it is important to limit sodium intake by avoiding high-sodium processed and packaged foods, using less salt in cooking and at the table, and paying attention to hidden sources of sodium in condiments, sauces, and snacks.

Protein intake: Diets that are high in animal protein, particularly from red meat, can increase the risk of kidney stone formation. Protein metabolism can lead to increased production of uric acid and other substances that can contribute to stone formation. Therefore, it is recommended to consume moderate amounts of high-quality protein from lean meats, poultry, fish, eggs, beans, and legumes, and limit intake of red meat and processed meats.

Fruit and vegetable intake: Diets rich in fruits and vegetables, particularly those high in potassium, citrate, and magnesium, have been associated with a reduced risk of kidney stone formation. These nutrients can help prevent the formation of certain types of kidney stones and promote overall kidney health. Good dietary sources of these nutrients include oranges, bananas, melons, leafy greens, broccoli, sweet potatoes, and beans.

Acidic and sugary foods and beverages: Diets that are high in acidic and sugary foods and beverages can also contribute to kidney stone formation. Excessive consumption of foods and beverages that are high in added sugars, such as soft drinks, energy drinks, candies, and desserts, can lead to increased urinary excretion of calcium and oxalate, which can promote stone formation.

Similarly, diets that are high in acidic foods, such as citrus fruits, tomatoes, vinegar, and acidic beverages, can increase the risk of uric acid stone formation in susceptible individuals. It is important to consume these foods and beverages in moderation and balance them with other healthy dietary choices.

Vitamin and mineral supplements: Taking excessive amounts of certain vitamin and mineral supplements, such as vitamin C and vitamin D, can increase the risk of kidney stone formation. Vitamin C is converted to oxalate in the body, and high doses of vitamin C supplements can lead to increased oxalate levels in urine.

Alongside, excessive vitamin D intake can increase the absorption of calcium in the gut, leading to increased urinary calcium excretion and potentially contributing to stone formation. It is important to talk to a healthcare professional before taking any vitamin or mineral supplements, especially in high doses.

Overall dietary pattern: In addition to individual nutrients and foods, the overall dietary pattern also plays a role in kidney stone prevention. Following a balanced and healthy diet, such as the

DASH (Dietary Approaches to Stop Hypertension) diet or the Mediterranean diet, which emphasize whole grains, fruits, vegetables, lean proteins, and healthy fats, can help reduce the risk of kidney stone formation. These diets are generally low in sodium, high in potassium, and promote overall kidney health.

Individual factors: It is important to note that the impact of diet on kidney stone formation can vary depending on individual factors such as age, gender, body weight, medical history, and genetic predisposition. Therefore, it is essential to work with a healthcare professional, such as a registered dietitian or a urologist, to determine the most appropriate dietary recommendations for each individual's unique needs and health status.

Goals of a kidney stone diet

The goals of a kidney stone diet are centered on reducing the risk of kidney stone formation, managing underlying medical conditions that may contribute to stone formation, and promoting overall kidney health. The specific goals of a kidney stone diet may vary depending on the type, size, location, and composition of the stones, as well as the individual's medical history, lifestyle, and dietary preferences.

Preventing stone formation: The primary goal of a kidney stone diet is to prevent the formation of new stones. This may involve dietary modifications to reduce the intake of substances that can contribute to stone formation, such as oxalate, calcium, and certain foods or beverages.

For example, a diet low in oxalate may be recommended for individuals with calcium oxalate stones, which are the most common type of kidney stones. Limiting the intake of high-oxalate foods, such as spinach, beets, nuts, chocolate, and certain beverages like tea and coffee, can help reduce the risk of calcium oxalate stone formation.

Promoting proper hydration: Staying well-hydrated is crucial in preventing kidney stone formation. Adequate fluid intake helps to increase urine volume and dilute the concentration of minerals and salts in the urine, reducing the risk of stone formation. The type and amount of fluids recommended may vary depending on factors such as the individual's body weight, climate, physical activity level, and medical history.

Water is typically the best choice for hydration, but other fluids such as herbal tea, diluted fruit juices, and clear soups may also be included in the diet. Avoiding sugary beverages, caffeinated beverages, and excessive alcohol consumption is also recommended as they can increase the risk of stone formation.

Managing underlying medical conditions: If an individual has underlying medical conditions that contribute to kidney stone formation, such as hyperparathyroidism, cystinuria, or renal tubular acidosis, the kidney stone diet may also aim to manage these conditions. This may involve working closely with a healthcare professional to develop a dietary plan that addresses the specific needs of the individual's medical condition.

For example, individuals with hyperparathyroidism may need to limit their intake of calcium-rich foods, while those with cystinuria may need to follow a low-cystine diet.

Balancing nutrient intake: A kidney stone diet should aim to provide a well-balanced intake of essential nutrients while avoiding excessive intake of substances that can contribute to stone formation. This may involve working with a registered dietitian or healthcare professional to develop a customized meal plan that meets the individual's nutrient needs.

For example, ensuring adequate intake of calcium from dietary sources is important, as a low-calcium diet can actually increase the risk of kidney stone formation. However, the type and amount of dietary calcium may need to be tailored based on the individual's specific type of stones and medical history.

Encouraging healthy eating habits: A kidney stone diet should also promote healthy eating habits that can support overall kidney health. This may involve consuming a diet that is rich in fruits, vegetables, whole grains, lean proteins, and healthy fats, while limiting processed foods, sugary foods, and excessive salt intake. Maintaining a healthy body weight, engaging in regular physical activity, and avoiding tobacco and excessive alcohol consumption can also support overall kidney health and reduce the risk of kidney stone formation.

Educating and empowering individuals: Another important goal of a kidney stone diet is to educate and empower individuals to make informed dietary choices and lifestyle changes to prevent stone formation. This may involve providing education on the importance of proper hydration, the impact of different foods and beverages on kidney stone formation, and strategies for managing underlying medical conditions. Providing practical tips for meal planning, grocery shopping, cooking, and dining out can also empower individuals to make healthier choices and adhere to their kidney stone diet plan.

Monitoring progress and adjusting the diet plan: Regular monitoring of progress and adjustments to the kidney stone diet plan may be necessary to optimize outcomes. This may involve regular follow-up appointments with a healthcare professional or registered dietitian to assess the effectiveness of the diet plan, review any changes in medical history or lifestyle factors, and make necessary adjustments to the diet plan based on individual needs and goals. Monitoring urinary parameters, such as urine volume, pH, and specific gravity, may also be recommended to assess the effectiveness of the diet plan in reducing the risk of stone formation.

Enhancing long-term kidney health: In addition to preventing kidney stone formation, a kidney stone diet should also aim to promote long-term kidney health. This may involve providing adequate nutrients that support kidney function, such as antioxidants, vitamins, and minerals, while avoiding excessive intake of substances that can damage the kidneys, such as high doses of certain supplements or medications. Promoting overall heart health, managing blood pressure and blood sugar levels, and avoiding tobacco and excessive alcohol consumption are also important for maintaining long-term kidney health and reducing the risk of kidney stone formation.

In summary, the goals of a kidney stone diet are multi-faceted and include preventing stone formation, promoting proper hydration, managing underlying medical conditions, balancing nutrient intake, encouraging healthy eating habits, educating and empowering individuals, monitoring progress, and enhancing long-term kidney health.

Working closely with a healthcare professional or registered dietitian can help individuals develop a comprehensive and personalized kidney stone diet plan that aligns with your specific needs and goals, and supports overall kidney health.

CHAPTER 2: THE KIDNEY STONE DIET: MACRONUTRIENTS AND MICRONUTRIENTS

Carbohydrates, proteins, and fats in a kidney stone diet

Carbohydrates, proteins, and fats are essential macronutrients that play a significant role in our diet and overall health. When it comes to a kidney stone diet, understanding how these macronutrients can affect kidney stone formation and incorporating appropriate dietary modifications can be crucial in preventing stone formation and managing kidney stone risk.

Carbohydrates:

Carbohydrates are an important source of energy for our bodies and can be found in various foods, such as grains, fruits, vegetables, and dairy products. In a kidney stone diet, it is recommended to choose complex carbohydrates, which are rich in fiber and provide sustained energy, rather than simple carbohydrates that are high in added sugars. Foods that are high in added sugars, such as sugary beverages, candies, and desserts, can increase the risk of kidney stone formation as they can lead to increased urine sugar levels and alter urinary composition.

Fiber-rich carbohydrates, such as whole grains, fruits, and vegetables, are beneficial for kidney stone prevention. Fiber helps in reducing the absorption of certain minerals, including calcium and oxalate, from the digestive tract, which can help in preventing the formation of calcium oxalate stones, the most common type of kidney stones.

Additionally, fiber promotes regular bowel movements, which can help in flushing out waste products and preventing the accumulation of stone-forming substances in the body.

Proteins:

Proteins are important for building and repairing tissues, maintaining muscle mass, and supporting various physiological functions in the body. However, certain sources and excessive intake of proteins can increase the risk of kidney stone formation. Animal-based proteins, such as meat, fish, and poultry, are high in purines, which are converted into uric acid in the body. High levels of uric acid in the urine can contribute to the formation of uric acid stones, which are another common type of kidney stones.

It is recommended to choose lean protein sources, such as poultry, fish, beans, legumes, and tofu, over high-purine animal-based proteins to reduce the risk of uric acid stone formation. Moderation in protein intake is also important, as excessive protein intake can lead to increased urinary excretion of calcium, oxalate, and uric acid, which can contribute to the formation of kidney stones.

Fats:

Fats are an essential component of our diet and are necessary for various physiological functions, such as hormone production, nutrient absorption, and energy storage. However, not all fats are created equal, and certain types of fats can impact kidney stone risk.

Saturated fats, which are commonly found in animal-based products, processed foods, and tropical oils, can increase the risk of kidney stone formation by increasing urinary calcium excretion and promoting oxidative stress. It is recommended to limit the intake of saturated fats in a kidney stone diet.

On the other hand, unsaturated fats, such as monounsaturated fats and polyunsaturated fats, found in foods like nuts, seeds, avocados, fatty fish, and olive oil, are considered healthy fats and can be beneficial in a kidney stone diet. These fats can help in reducing inflammation, promoting heart health, and improving overall well-being.

In a wrap, a well-balanced kidney stone diet should focus on incorporating complex carbohydrates, lean protein sources, and healthy fats while limiting simple carbohydrates, high-purine animal-based proteins, and saturated fats. Staying hydrated and maintaining a healthy weight through regular physical activity and lifestyle modifications are also crucial in preventing kidney stone formation.

Recommended intake and sources of fiber

Fiber is an essential nutrient that plays a crucial role in maintaining good overall health, including digestive health, heart health, and weight management. A diet rich in fiber has been associated with numerous health benefits, including improved digestion, lowered risk of chronic diseases such as cardiovascular disease, diabetes, and certain types of cancer, and better weight management.

Recommended Intake of Fiber:

The recommended daily intake of fiber varies depending on age, sex, and activity level. According to the Dietary Guidelines for Americans, the recommended daily fiber intake for adults is as follows:

- For men: 38 grams of fiber per day.
- For women: 25 grams of fiber per day for those under 50 years of age, and 21 grams per day for those over 50 years of age.

It is important to note that these are general recommendations, and individual needs may vary. It is always best to consult with a healthcare professional or a registered dietitian for personalized dietary recommendations.

Sources of Fiber:

Fiber can be found in a wide variety of plant-based foods, including fruits, vegetables, whole grains, legumes, nuts, and seeds. Here are some examples of high-fiber foods:

Fruits: Many fruits are good sources of fiber. Berries, apples, oranges, bananas, pears, and avocados are some examples of fruits that are high in fiber. It is recommended to eat fruits with the skin on, whenever possible, as the skin is often a good source of fiber.

Vegetables: Vegetables are rich in fiber and should be an important part of a high-fiber diet. Leafy greens, broccoli, Brussels sprouts, carrots, sweet potatoes, and artichokes are some examples of high-fiber vegetables.

Whole grains: Whole grains are an excellent source of dietary fiber. Brown rice, quinoa, oats, whole wheat, whole grain bread, and whole grain pasta are some examples of whole grain foods that are high in fiber. When choosing grains, it's important to look for "whole" grains in the ingredient list, as refined grains may have less fiber.

Legumes: Legumes, including beans, lentils, chickpeas, and peas, are rich in fiber, protein, and other important nutrients. Adding legumes to soups, stews, salads, and side dishes can easily boost the fiber content of your meals.

Nuts and seeds: Nuts and seeds are a great source of fiber, healthy fats, and other essential nutrients. Almonds, chia seeds, flaxseeds, and sunflower seeds are some examples of nuts and seeds that are high in fiber. They can be added to smoothies, yogurt, salads, or eaten as a snack.

Other sources: Some other foods that are good sources of fiber include popcorn, bran cereals, and whole grain crackers. It's important to read food labels and choose products that are high in fiber.

Incorporating Fiber into Your Diet:

Here are some tips on how to incorporate more fiber into your diet:

Eat whole foods: Choose whole, unprocessed foods as much as possible. Whole fruits and vegetables, whole grains, legumes, nuts, and seeds are all great sources of fiber.

Eat a variety of fiber-rich foods: Different types of fiber have different health benefits, so it's important to eat a variety of fiber-rich foods. Include a mix of fruits, vegetables, whole grains, legumes, nuts, and seeds in your diet.

Gradually increase fiber intake: If you are not used to a high-fiber diet, it's important to gradually increase your fiber intake to avoid digestive discomfort. Start by adding small amounts of fiber-rich foods to your diet and gradually increase the amount over time, while also drinking plenty of water to help with digestion.

Choose whole grains: When choosing grains, opt for whole grains over refined grains. Whole grains are higher in fiber and other important nutrients, as they contain the entire grain, including the bran, germ, and endosperm.

Include fruits and vegetables in every meal: Aim to have fruits and vegetables in every meal and snack. They can be incorporated in a variety of ways, such as in salads, soups, stir-fries, smoothies, or as snacks.

Snack on nuts and seeds: Nuts and seeds make for a healthy and convenient high-fiber snack. Keep a stash of almonds, chia seeds, or sunflower seeds on hand for a quick and satisfying snack.

Add legumes to your meals: Legumes, such as beans, lentils, and chickpeas, are versatile and can be added to soups, stews, salads, and side dishes to increase the fiber content of your meals.

Be mindful of food preparation methods: Opt for cooking methods that retain the fiber content of foods, such as steaming, roasting, or baking, instead of deep frying or boiling.

Read food labels: When shopping for packaged foods, read the nutrition labels and choose products that are high in fiber. Look for foods with at least 3 grams of fiber per serving.

Seek guidance from a healthcare professional or registered dietitian: If you have specific dietary needs or health conditions, it's helpful to seek guidance from a healthcare professional or registered dietitian to determine the right amount and sources of fiber for your individual needs.

Incorporating fiber-rich foods into your diet is essential for maintaining good overall health, including digestive health. Aim to consume a variety of high-fiber foods, such as fruits, vegetables, whole grains, legumes, nuts, and seeds, and gradually increase your fiber intake over time.

Remember to drink plenty of water and consult with a healthcare professional or registered dietitian for personalized dietary recommendations.

Role of calcium, sodium, potassium, and magnesium in kidney stone prevention

Kidney stones, also known as renal calculi, are solid masses that form in the kidneys from the accumulation of various substances. Calcium, sodium, potassium, and magnesium are essential minerals that play important roles in the prevention of kidney stones. Understanding their roles can help in the management and prevention of kidney stones.

Calcium:

Calcium is a crucial mineral that is necessary for numerous bodily functions, including bone and teeth formation, nerve function, muscle function, and blood clotting. However, calcium is also a common component of kidney stones, with calcium-containing stones accounting for approximately 80% of all kidney stones. It is important to note that calcium from food sources does not increase the risk of kidney stones, but rather, it is excessive calcium supplementation or high intake of calcium-rich foods that may contribute to stone formation.

Calcium also interacts with other substances in the urinary tract, such as oxalate and phosphate, to form insoluble crystals that can precipitate and result in stone formation. However, calcium also has a preventive role in kidney stone formation, as it can bind to oxalate in the intestines, reducing its absorption and decreasing the amount of oxalate that is excreted in the urine, thus reducing the risk of calcium-oxalate stone formation.

Sodium:

Sodium is another mineral that can impact kidney stone formation. Diets high in sodium can lead to increased urinary excretion of calcium, which can raise the risk of kidney stone formation. Sodium can also lead to increased water retention, resulting in reduced urine output and concentrated urine, which can increase the risk of stone formation. Therefore, reducing sodium intake, especially from processed foods and table salt, is recommended for kidney stone prevention.

Potassium:

Potassium is an essential mineral that is vital for maintaining proper fluid and electrolyte balance in the body. It can counteract the negative effects of sodium by promoting diuresis and increasing urine output, which helps to flush out stone-forming substances from the kidneys.

Additionally, potassium has been shown to reduce the excretion of calcium in the urine, which can further lower the risk of calcium-containing stone formation. Including potassium-rich foods such as bananas, oranges, spinach, and sweet potatoes in the diet can be beneficial for kidney stone prevention.

Magnesium:

Magnesium is a mineral that plays a role in many enzymatic reactions in the body and is known to inhibit the formation of calcium-oxalate crystals, which are the most common type of kidney stones. Magnesium can also bind to oxalate in the gastrointestinal tract, reducing its absorption and excretion in the urine. Adequate intake of magnesium through a balanced diet that includes whole grains, nuts, seeds, legumes, and leafy green vegetables can help in the prevention of kidney stones.

In addition to the roles of calcium, sodium, potassium, and magnesium in kidney stone prevention, it is important to maintain proper hydration by drinking an adequate amount of water throughout the day. Sufficient water intake helps to dilute urine, reducing the concentration of stone-forming substances and preventing their precipitation. A general guideline is to drink at least 8-10 glasses of water per day, but individual requirements may vary depending on factors such as climate, physical activity level, and medical conditions.

Other essential vitamins and minerals

In addition to calcium, sodium, potassium, and magnesium, there are several other essential vitamins and minerals that play important roles in kidney stone prevention:

Vitamin B6 (Pyridoxine): Vitamin B6 is known to reduce the production of oxalate in the body, which is a common component of kidney stones. Adequate intake of vitamin B6 through a balanced diet that includes poultry, fish, bananas, avocados, and nuts can help in preventing the formation of calcium-oxalate stones.

Vitamin D: Vitamin D is essential for calcium absorption and bone health. However, excessive intake of vitamin D supplements can lead to increased levels of calcium in the blood and urine, increasing the risk of calcium-containing kidney stones. It is important to maintain appropriate levels of vitamin D, as recommended by healthcare professionals, to prevent kidney stone formation.

Vitamin K: Vitamin K is involved in calcium regulation in the body and can help prevent the formation of calcium-oxalate stones. Good dietary sources of vitamin K include leafy green vegetables, broccoli, Brussels sprouts, and fermented foods.

Phosphorus: Phosphorus is an essential mineral that works with calcium to build and maintain strong bones and teeth. However, excessive intake of phosphorus, often found in processed foods and sodas, can lead to increased urinary excretion of calcium, increasing the risk of kidney stone formation. Balancing phosphorus intake with calcium intake is important for kidney stone prevention.

Citrate: Citrate is a natural inhibitor of stone formation as it can bind to calcium and prevent the formation of calcium crystals. Citrate is naturally found in citrus fruits like oranges and lemons, and its intake can help in preventing the formation of calcium-containing stones.

Oxalate: While oxalate is a common component of kidney stones, adequate intake of dietary oxalate can actually help in preventing kidney stone formation. This is because oxalate can bind to calcium in the intestines, reducing its absorption and excretion in the urine. Foods that are high in oxalate include spinach, beets, sweet potatoes, nuts, and tea.

Fluids: Maintaining proper hydration is crucial for kidney stone prevention. Sufficient water intake helps to flush out stone-forming substances from the kidneys and dilutes the urine, reducing the concentration of stone-forming substances. In addition to water, herbal teas, and other non-sugary beverages can also contribute to proper hydration.

It is important to note that the optimal intake of these vitamins and minerals for kidney stone prevention may vary depending on an individual's health status, age, sex, and other factors.

CHAPTER 3: FOOD GROUPS AND KIDNEY STONE PREVENTION

Kidney stone prevention involves not only paying attention to specific nutrients, but also adopting a balanced diet that includes a variety of food groups. Here are some key considerations for each food group in relation to kidney stone prevention:

Whole grains and legumes:

Whole grains, such as brown rice, quinoa, and whole wheat bread, are rich in fiber, which can help regulate bowel movements and prevent constipation. Legumes, such as lentils, beans, and chickpeas, are also high in fiber and plant-based protein, which can promote overall digestive health and provide important nutrients for kidney stone prevention. Additionally, whole grains and legumes are typically low in oxalate, which is a common component of kidney stones, making them a healthy choice for kidney stone prevention.

Fruits and vegetables:

Fruits and vegetables are crucial components of a kidney stone prevention diet. They are rich in fiber, vitamins, minerals, and antioxidants, which can support overall health and help prevent kidney stone formation. Many fruits and vegetables are also low in oxalate, making them an excellent choice for individuals prone to kidney stones.

Citrus fruits, such as oranges and lemons, are particularly beneficial, as they are high in citrate, which can inhibit the formation of kidney stones. Other low-oxalate fruits and vegetables, such as apples, berries, cucumbers, bell peppers, and cauliflower, can also be included in the diet to promote kidney stone prevention.

Dairy products and alternatives:

Dairy products and their alternatives are important sources of calcium, which is a vital mineral for overall bone health. Calcium from food sources can actually help bind to oxalate in the gut, reducing the absorption of oxalate and lowering the risk of kidney stone formation. However, it is important to choose low-fat or non-fat options to avoid excessive intake of animal protein and high-fat dairy products, which can increase the risk of kidney stone formation. Good choices include low-fat milk, yogurt, and cheese, as well as plant-based alternatives like almond milk, soy milk, and tofu.

Meat and poultry:

Meat and poultry are rich sources of protein, but high intake of animal protein can increase the risk of kidney stone formation in some individuals. Animal protein can lead to increased urinary excretion of calcium, oxalate, and other substances that can contribute to kidney stone formation. Therefore, it is important to moderate the intake of meat and poultry and choose lean cuts whenever possible. Incorporating other sources of protein such as legumes, nuts, and seeds can also be beneficial in kidney stone prevention.

Seafood and fish:

Seafood and fish are excellent sources of omega-3 fatty acids, which have anti-inflammatory properties and can promote overall heart health. However, some types of fish, such as sardines, mackerel, and trout, can be high in purines, which can increase the risk of uric acid stones in susceptible individuals. Purines are broken down into uric acid in the body, and excessive uric acid can contribute to the formation of uric acid stones. It is important to consume fish and seafood in moderation and choose low-purine options like salmon, tuna, and shrimp.

Fats, oils, and sweets:

Fats, oils, and sweets should be consumed in moderation as part of a healthy kidney stone prevention diet. High intake of added sugars, saturated fats, and trans fats can contribute to weight gain, inflammation, and other health issues, which may increase the risk of kidney stone formation. Choosing healthier fats such as olive oil, avocado, and nuts, and limiting added sugars and unhealthy fats from processed foods, sweets, and desserts is recommended for kidney stone prevention.

In addition to food groups, there are other dietary considerations that can help prevent kidney stones. These include:

Adequate fluid intake: Staying well-hydrated is crucial in kidney stone prevention. It helps to dilute urine, flush out waste products, and prevent the formation of crystals that can lead to stone formation. Water is the best option for hydration, but other fluids like herbal tea, lemonade, and low-sugar fruit juices can also be included. Aim to drink at least 8-10 cups (64-80 ounces) of fluids per day, or more if you are physically active or live in a hot climate.

Moderation of high-oxalate foods: Oxalate is a common component of kidney stones, and some foods are high in oxalate. Examples of high-oxalate foods include spinach, beets, sweet potatoes, nuts, chocolate, and tea. While these foods can be part of a healthy diet, consuming them in excess may increase the risk of kidney stone formation in susceptible individuals. It's important to consume them in moderation and balance them with low-oxalate foods.

Limitation of sodium intake: High sodium intake can lead to increased urinary excretion of calcium, which can contribute to kidney stone formation. Therefore, it's important to limit the consumption of high-sodium foods such as processed foods, fast foods, canned foods, and salty snacks. Opt for low-sodium options and use herbs, spices, and other flavorings to season foods instead of salt.

Calcium intake from food sources: Calcium is an important mineral for overall bone health and can also play a role in kidney stone prevention. Consuming adequate amounts of calcium from food sources can actually help bind to oxalate in the gut, reducing its absorption and lowering the risk of kidney stone formation. Good sources of calcium include low-fat dairy products or alternatives, fortified plant-based milks, and calcium-rich foods like leafy greens, broccoli, and almonds.

Balanced protein intake: While protein is important for overall health, high intake of animal protein can increase the risk of kidney stone formation in some individuals. It's important to balance protein intake by incorporating a variety of protein sources such as legumes, nuts, seeds, and plant-based proteins along with moderate amounts of lean meat, poultry, and seafood.

Vitamin and mineral supplements: While it's best to obtain essential vitamins and minerals from whole foods, in some cases, supplementation may be necessary. Talk to your healthcare provider or a registered dietitian before taking any vitamin or mineral supplements, as excessive intake of certain supplements may increase the risk of kidney stone formation, especially if you have a history of kidney stones or other health conditions.

A well-balanced diet that includes whole grains and legumes, a variety of fruits and vegetables, low-fat dairy products or alternatives, lean meat and poultry, low purine seafood and fish, and moderate intake of fats, oils, and sweets can play an important role in kidney stone prevention. It is also essential to stay well-hydrated by drinking plenty of water throughout the day to flush out toxins and prevent the formation of kidney stones.

CHAPTER 4: KIDNEY STONE DIET RECIPES AND MEAL PLANS

Breakfast Recipes:

BLUEBERRY SPINACH SMOOTHIE

Ingredients:

- 1 cup frozen blueberries
- 1 cup fresh spinach
- 1 small banana, ripe
- 1/2 cup plain Greek yogurt
- 1 tbsp chia seeds
- 1/2 cup unsweetened almond milk (or any milk of your choice)
- 1 tsp honey (optional for sweetness)

Instructions:

- Add all the ingredients into a blender in the following order: frozen blueberries, fresh spinach, ripe banana, Greek yogurt, chia seeds, almond milk, and honey (if using).
- Blend on high speed until the mixture is smooth and creamy.
- Stop the blender and scrape down the sides if needed, then blend again until fully combined.
- Taste and adjust sweetness with honey, if desired.
- Pour into glasses and enjoy immediately as a refreshing smoothie!

Cooking Tips:

- Using frozen blueberries adds natural sweetness and makes the smoothie colder and thicker, but you can also use fresh blueberries if preferred.
- Ripe bananas are sweeter and easier to blend, so be sure to use a ripe banana in this recipe.
- Greek yogurt adds creaminess and protein to the smoothie, but you can use any type of plain yogurt or a dairy-free alternative if preferred.

- Chia seeds are optional, but they add fiber and healthy fats which can be beneficial for kidney stone prevention.
- Adjust the sweetness of the smoothie with honey or any other natural sweetener according to your preference.
- If you prefer a thinner consistency, you can add more almond milk or water to achieve your desired consistency.

VEGGIE OMELETTE WITH SPINACH AND MUSHROOMS

Ingredients:

- 2 large eggs
- 1/4 cup chopped spinach
- 1/4 cup sliced mushrooms
- 1/4 cup diced red bell pepper
- 1/4 cup crumbled feta cheese
- 1 tablespoon olive oil
- Salt and pepper to taste

Cooking Instructions:

- Heat a non-stick skillet over medium heat and add olive oil.

- Add the sliced mushrooms and diced red bell pepper to the skillet and sauté for 2-3 minutes until slightly softened.

- Add the chopped spinach to the skillet and sauté for another 1-2 minutes until wilted.

- In a separate bowl, whisk the eggs together with a pinch of salt and pepper.

- Pour the whisked eggs over the sautéed vegetables in the skillet.

- Allow the omelette to cook for 2-3 minutes until the edges are set and the middle is slightly runny.

- Sprinkle the crumbled feta cheese evenly over one half of the omelette.

- Using a spatula, fold the other half of the omelette over the cheese to form a half-moon shape.

- Cook for another 1-2 minutes until the cheese is melted and the omelette is cooked through.

- Slide the omelette onto a plate and serve hot.

Cooking Tips:

- Use a non-stick skillet to prevent the omelette from sticking and ensure easy flipping.

- Adjust the amount of salt and pepper to your taste preferences, keeping in mind any dietary restrictions or guidelines provided by your healthcare professional.

- You can also add other kidney stone-friendly vegetables such as asparagus, zucchini, or kale to the omelette for added nutrition.

- Avoid adding high-oxalate foods such as tomatoes, beets, or sweet potatoes, which can contribute to kidney stone formation, to this omelette recipe.

- Remember to stay hydrated and drink plenty of water throughout the day to support kidney health and prevent kidney stone formation.

QUINOA BREAKFAST BOWL WITH FRESH FRUIT

Ingredients:

- 1 cup quinoa
- 2 cups water
- 1/2 teaspoon cinnamon
- 1/2 teaspoon vanilla extract

- 1 tablespoon honey or maple syrup (optional, adjust to taste)
- 1/2 cup fresh mixed berries (such as blueberries, strawberries, raspberries)
- 1 small banana, sliced
- 1/4 cup chopped nuts (such as almonds, walnuts, or pecans)
- Fresh mint leaves for garnish (optional)

Cooking Instructions:

- Rinse the quinoa thoroughly under cold water in a fine-mesh strainer to remove any bitterness.
- In a saucepan, combine quinoa and water, and bring to a boil.
- Reduce heat to low, cover with a lid, and simmer for 15-20 minutes or until the quinoa is cooked and the water is absorbed.
- Remove from heat and let it sit covered for 5 minutes.
- Fluff the quinoa with a fork and stir in cinnamon, vanilla extract, and honey or maple syrup (if using).
- Allow the quinoa to cool slightly.
- In serving bowls, place a generous scoop of cooked quinoa.
- Top with fresh mixed berries, sliced banana, and chopped nuts.
- Garnish with fresh mint leaves (if using).

- Serve warm and enjoy!

Cooking Tips:

- For individuals with kidney stones, it's important to monitor the portion size of foods high in oxalates, such as nuts and berries. If you have a history of calcium oxalate stones, you may want to limit the amount of high-oxalate foods in your diet.

- Be sure to rinse the quinoa thoroughly before cooking to remove the bitter coating called saponin.

- Adjust the sweetness of the breakfast bowl by adding honey or maple syrup to your liking. However, if you have diabetes or need to watch your sugar intake, you may want to skip or reduce the sweetener.

- You can also customize this breakfast bowl by adding other kidney-friendly fruits, such as diced apples or sliced peaches, and swapping nuts for seeds like sunflower seeds or flaxseeds.

- Fresh mint leaves can add a refreshing flavor to the bowl, but they are optional. Feel free to omit them if you prefer.

GREEK YOGURT PARFAIT WITH BERRIES AND NUTS

Ingredients:

- 1 cup plain Greek yogurt (low-fat or non-fat)
- 1 cup mixed berries (such as blueberries, strawberries, raspberries)
- 1/4 cup chopped nuts (such as almonds, walnuts, or pistachios)
- 1 tbsp honey (optional)
- 1/2 tsp cinnamon (optional)

Cooking Instructions:

- Wash and prepare the berries by removing stems and hulls, if necessary. You can use fresh or frozen berries depending on your preference and availability.
- In a separate bowl, mix the Greek yogurt with honey (if using) and cinnamon (if using) to sweeten and flavor the yogurt to your liking.
- Layer the Greek yogurt, berries, and chopped nuts in a serving glass or bowl, starting with a layer of yogurt, followed by a layer of berries, and a sprinkle of nuts. Repeat the layers until all the ingredients are used up.

- Optionally, you can drizzle additional honey on top for added sweetness, and sprinkle some cinnamon for extra flavor.
- Serve and enjoy your kidney stone-friendly Greek Yogurt Parfait with Berries and Nuts!

Cooking Tips:

- Greek yogurt is a good source of protein, calcium, and probiotics, which can help support overall kidney health. Opt for plain Greek yogurt without added sugars or flavors for a healthier option.
- Berries are rich in antioxidants, fiber, and vitamins, which can promote overall health and may help prevent kidney stone formation. Choose a variety of berries for added nutrition.
- Nuts, such as almonds, walnuts, or pistachios, can add crunch and healthy fats to your parfait. These nuts are also rich in magnesium, which is known to help prevent kidney stones. Choose unsalted nuts for a lower sodium option.
- You can customize the sweetness and flavor of your parfait by adding honey and cinnamon, but be mindful of your sugar intake, especially if you have diabetes or other health conditions. Use them sparingly or omit them if desired.

AVOCADO AND EGG TOAST

Ingredients:

- 1 ripe avocado
- 2 eggs
- 2 slices of whole grain bread
- 1 small tomato, diced
- Fresh cilantro or parsley, chopped (optional)
- Salt and pepper, to taste

Cooking Instructions:

- Toast the slices of whole grain bread in a toaster or on a stovetop griddle until crispy.
- Meanwhile, halve the ripe avocado, remove the pit, and scoop out the flesh into a bowl. Mash the avocado with a fork or a potato masher until it reaches your desired consistency.
- In a small saucepan, bring water to a gentle simmer. Crack each egg into a separate ramekin or small bowl. Carefully slide each egg into the simmering water and cook for about

3-4 minutes until the whites are set but the yolks are still slightly runny.

- Remove the poached eggs from the water with a slotted spoon and place them on a paper towel-lined plate to drain any excess water.
- Spread the mashed avocado onto the toasted bread slices. Top with diced tomatoes and a sprinkle of salt and pepper.
- Gently place a poached egg on top of each avocado toast.
- Garnish with fresh cilantro or parsley, if desired.
- Serve and enjoy!

Cooking Tips:

- Use ripe avocados for the best flavor and texture. Look for avocados that yield slightly to gentle pressure when pressed with your fingers, but are not overly soft or mushy.
- Whole grain bread is a healthier option compared to refined grains, as it contains more fiber and nutrients. Look for bread with minimal added sugars and preservatives for a kidney stone-friendly option.
- Be careful when poaching eggs to avoid overcooking them. Aim for a slightly runny yolk, as overcooked yolks can become hard and less appealing.

- You can also customize this recipe by adding other kidney stone-friendly ingredients such as chopped leafy greens, diced cucumber, or crumbled feta cheese for added flavor and nutrition.

BERRY CHIA SEED PUDDING

Ingredients:

- 1/2 cup chia seeds
- 2 cups unsweetened almond milk (or any milk of your choice)
- 1 tsp pure vanilla extract
- 1 tbsp honey (or sweetener of your choice)
- 1 cup mixed berries (such as blueberries, strawberries, raspberries)
- 1 tbsp chopped nuts (such as almonds or walnuts) for garnish (optional)

Cooking Instructions:

- In a mixing bowl, whisk together chia seeds, almond milk, vanilla extract, and honey (or sweetener) until well combined.
- Let the mixture sit for about 5 minutes, then whisk again to prevent clumping.
- Cover the bowl and refrigerate the chia seed mixture for at least 4 hours or overnight, allowing it to thicken into a pudding-like consistency.
- Before serving, give the chia seed pudding a good stir to ensure even distribution of the chia seeds.
- Wash and prepare the mixed berries by washing them thoroughly and removing any stems or leaves. Slice strawberries if desired.
- To serve, spoon the chilled chia seed pudding into serving bowls or glasses.
- Top the chia seed pudding with the mixed berries and garnish with chopped nuts, if desired.
- Enjoy the delicious and nutritious Berry Chia Seed Pudding as a healthy dessert or breakfast option!

Cooking Tips:

- Adjust the sweetness to your preference by using more or less honey or sweetener.

- You can use any type of milk (such as almond milk, coconut milk, or cow's milk) that suits your dietary needs and preferences.

- Make sure to stir the chia seed mixture after the initial 5 minutes of soaking to prevent clumping and ensure a smooth consistency.

- Allow the chia seed pudding to refrigerate for at least 4 hours or overnight for best results, as this allows the chia seeds to fully absorb the liquid and thicken.

- Feel free to customize the mixed berries based on what's in season or what you have available. Berries are generally a good choice for kidney stone prevention due to their high water content and antioxidants.

- Nuts can add a crunchy texture and healthy fats to the chia seed pudding, but they are optional and can be omitted if you have nut allergies or other dietary restrictions.

SWEET POTATO HASH WITH KALE AND EGGS

Ingredients:

- 1 large sweet potato, peeled and diced into small cubes
- 1 small red onion, finely chopped

- 2 cloves garlic, minced
- 2 cups kale, stems removed and chopped
- 4 large eggs
- 2 tablespoons olive oil
- 1 teaspoon paprika
- Salt and pepper to taste
- Optional: chopped fresh herbs (such as parsley or cilantro) for garnish

Cooking Instructions:

- Heat a large skillet over medium heat and add the olive oil.
- Add the diced sweet potatoes to the skillet and cook for 5-7 minutes, stirring occasionally, until they start to soften.
- Add the chopped red onion and minced garlic to the skillet with the sweet potatoes and cook for another 2-3 minutes until the onion is translucent.
- Stir in the chopped kale and paprika, and cook for another 2-3 minutes until the kale is wilted.
- Make four wells in the sweet potato hash mixture and crack an egg into each well.

- Reduce the heat to low, cover the skillet, and let the eggs cook for 5-7 minutes, or until the whites are set but the yolks are still slightly runny.
- Season the dish with salt and pepper to taste, and garnish with fresh herbs, if desired.
- Serve hot and enjoy!

Cooking Tips:

- To make the sweet potato hash cook faster, you can parboil the diced sweet potatoes for a few minutes before adding them to the skillet. This will help soften them and reduce the cooking time in the skillet.
- You can customize the seasoning in the dish by adding other kidney stone-friendly herbs and spices, such as thyme, rosemary, or turmeric, which are known for their anti-inflammatory properties.
- Be careful not to overcook the eggs, as they can become too firm and lose their runny yolk, which is part of the appeal of this dish. Keep an eye on the eggs while they are cooking and adjust the timing to your preference.
- This recipe can be easily modified to suit dietary preferences or restrictions. For example, you can use coconut oil instead

of olive oil for a different flavor profile, or swap kale with spinach or Swiss chard if preferred.

GREEN SMOOTHIE BOWL WITH KALE, BANANA, AND ALMOND MILK

Ingredients:

- 2 cups chopped kale leaves, stems removed
- 1 ripe banana, peeled and sliced
- 1 cup unsweetened almond milk
- 1 tablespoon chia seeds
- 1 tablespoon almond butter
- 1 teaspoon honey (optional)
- Ice (optional)

Cooking Instructions:

- Wash and thoroughly rinse the kale leaves, removing the tough stems.
- In a blender, combine the kale, banana, almond milk, chia seeds, almond butter, and honey (if using).

- Blend on high speed until the mixture is smooth and creamy, adding ice if desired for a colder consistency.
- Pour the green smoothie into a bowl.

Cooking Tips:

- If you prefer a sweeter smoothie, you can add more honey or a natural sweetener of your choice, such as maple syrup or agave nectar.
- To make the smoothie bowl thicker, you can add more ice or reduce the amount of almond milk.
- You can also customize this recipe by adding other kidney-friendly ingredients such as low-potassium fruits like berries or apples, and adjusting the recipe according to your dietary needs and preferences.

Kidney Stone-Friendly Optimization:

- This recipe uses kale, which is a low-oxalate leafy green vegetable that is less likely to contribute to oxalate-based kidney stones.
- Almond milk is a good alternative to dairy milk for individuals with lactose intolerance or those who prefer a

dairy-free option. It is also lower in phosphorus compared to cow's milk, which can be beneficial for kidney health.

- Chia seeds are a good source of fiber and healthy fats, and they are low in oxalates, making them a suitable addition to a kidney-friendly diet.
- Almond butter is a good source of healthy fats and protein, and it can add creaminess and flavor to the smoothie bowl.
- Honey is optional and can be used sparingly as a natural sweetener. However, it is important to keep in mind that excessive sugar intake should be avoided in a kidney-friendly diet, so use it in moderation or omit it if desired.

BUCKWHEAT PANCAKES WITH FRESH BERRIES

Ingredients:

- 1 cup buckwheat flour
- 1/2 cup almond flour
- 1/4 cup ground flaxseed
- 1 teaspoon baking powder
- 1/2 teaspoon baking soda
- 1/4 teaspoon salt
- 1 teaspoon cinnamon

- 1 ripe banana, mashed
- 2 large eggs
- 1 cup unsweetened almond milk (or any milk of your choice)
- 1 tablespoon honey (optional)
- Fresh berries (such as blueberries, strawberries, raspberries) for topping

Cooking Instructions:

- In a large mixing bowl, whisk together the buckwheat flour, almond flour, ground flaxseed, baking powder, baking soda, salt, and cinnamon.
- In a separate bowl, mash the ripe banana with a fork until smooth. Add the eggs, almond milk, and honey (if using) to the mashed banana and whisk until well combined.
- Pour the wet ingredients into the dry ingredients and stir until just combined, being careful not to overmix. The batter should be thick but pourable. If it's too thick, you can add a little more almond milk to achieve the desired consistency.
- Heat a non-stick skillet or griddle over medium heat and lightly grease with cooking spray or a little oil.
- Scoop 1/4 cup of the batter onto the hot skillet and spread it into a circle using the back of a spoon or a spatula.

- Cook for 2-3 minutes, until bubbles form on the surface of the pancake and the edges start to look set. Flip the pancake and cook for another 1-2 minutes until golden brown.
- Repeat with the remaining batter, adding a little more oil or cooking spray as needed to prevent sticking.
- Serve the buckwheat pancakes hot, topped with fresh berries.

Cooking Tips:

- Buckwheat flour and almond flour are good choices for kidney stone prevention as they are low in oxalate, which is a common component of kidney stones. Flaxseed is also a good source of dietary fiber and healthy fats.
- Mash the banana well to ensure it is fully blended into the batter and provides natural sweetness to the pancakes. You can adjust the amount of honey or sweetener to your taste preference.
- Avoid overmixing the batter to prevent tough pancakes. Stir until just combined for light and fluffy pancakes.
- Use a non-stick skillet or griddle and grease it lightly to prevent sticking and ensure even cooking.
- Top the pancakes with fresh berries, which are rich in antioxidants and nutrients, and can be beneficial for overall health, including kidney stone prevention.

SPINACH AND MUSHROOM FRITTATA

Ingredients:

- 6 large eggs
- 1 cup fresh spinach, chopped
- 1/2 cup mushrooms, sliced
- 1/4 cup red bell pepper, diced
- 1/4 cup red onion, diced
- 1/4 cup shredded low-fat cheese (such as mozzarella or Swiss)
- 2 tablespoons olive oil
- 1/2 teaspoon salt
- 1/4 teaspoon black pepper
- Cooking spray (optional)

Instructions:

- Preheat your oven to 350°F (175°C).
- In a medium-sized mixing bowl, whisk the eggs together with salt and black pepper.
- Heat olive oil in an oven-safe skillet over medium heat.

- Add the red onion and red bell pepper to the skillet and sauté for 2-3 minutes until they begin to soften.
- Add the mushrooms and cook for another 2-3 minutes until they start to release their moisture.
- Add the chopped spinach to the skillet and cook until wilted, about 1-2 minutes.
- Pour the whisked eggs evenly over the vegetables in the skillet.
- Sprinkle the shredded cheese on top.
- Cook the frittata on the stovetop for 3-4 minutes, until the edges are set but the center is still slightly runny.
- Transfer the skillet to the preheated oven and bake for 12-15 minutes, until the center is fully set and the top is lightly golden.
- Remove from the oven and let it cool for a few minutes.
- Cut into wedges and serve hot.

Cooking Tips:

- You can use a non-stick skillet or a cast-iron skillet for this recipe. If using a cast-iron skillet, make sure it is properly seasoned to prevent sticking.

- If you want to add more kidney-friendly ingredients, you can consider adding chopped fresh herbs like parsley or dill, or even some diced tomatoes for added flavor and nutrition.
- Avoid using excessive salt or high-sodium ingredients in the frittata, as a high-sodium diet can contribute to kidney stone formation. Use salt in moderation and choose low-sodium or salt-free options whenever possible.
- Cooking the frittata in the oven allows for even cooking and prevents the bottom from getting too browned. Make sure to use an oven-safe skillet if transferring to the oven.
- You can also use a cooking spray to coat the skillet before adding the vegetables to prevent sticking, if desired.

BREAKFAST BURRITO WITH BLACK BEANS, AVOCADO, AND SALSA

Ingredients:

4 large eggs

1 tablespoon olive oil

1/4 cup chopped red onion

1/2 cup canned black beans, drained and rinsed

1 small avocado, peeled, pitted, and diced

1/2 cup salsa (choose a low-sodium variety)

Salt and pepper to taste

4 whole wheat tortillas (8-inch diameter)

Chopped fresh cilantro (optional, for garnish)

Cooking Instructions:

- Heat olive oil in a non-stick skillet over medium heat.
- Add chopped red onion and cook until softened, about 2-3 minutes.
- Add black beans to the skillet and cook for another 2-3 minutes, stirring occasionally.
- In a separate bowl, whisk the eggs with a pinch of salt and pepper.
- Add the whisked eggs to the skillet with the black beans and onion, stirring gently until the eggs are fully cooked.
- Stir in diced avocado and salsa, and cook for another minute, until warmed through.
- Warm the whole wheat tortillas in a separate skillet or in the oven for a few seconds.

- Place a scoop of the egg and black bean mixture onto each tortilla.
- Fold the tortilla into a burrito shape, tucking in the sides as you roll.
- Garnish with chopped cilantro (optional).
- Serve hot and enjoy your kidney-friendly Breakfast Burrito!

Cooking Tips:

- You can adjust the amount of salsa to your preference, and choose a low-sodium variety to reduce sodium intake.
- Use whole wheat tortillas for added fiber and nutrients.
- Opt for a non-stick skillet to minimize the need for excess oil during cooking.
- Season with herbs and spices instead of salt to lower sodium content.
- You can also add other kidney-friendly ingredients such as bell peppers, tomatoes, or spinach to enhance the nutritional value of the burrito.

OATMEAL WITH FRESH FRUIT AND ALMONDS

Ingredients:

- 1 cup of rolled oats
- 2 cups of water
- 1/4 teaspoon of salt
- 1/2 teaspoon of cinnamon
- 1/2 teaspoon of vanilla extract
- 1/2 cup of mixed fresh fruits (such as berries, sliced banana, diced apple, or chopped peach)
- 2 tablespoons of chopped almonds
- 1 tablespoon of honey or maple syrup (optional)

Cooking Instructions:

- In a medium saucepan, combine the rolled oats, water, salt, cinnamon, and vanilla extract. Bring to a boil over medium heat, then reduce the heat to low and simmer for about 5 minutes, stirring occasionally, until the oats are creamy and tender.
- Remove the saucepan from heat and stir in the mixed fresh fruits and chopped almonds.
- Cover the saucepan and let the oatmeal stand for a couple of minutes to allow the fruits to soften slightly.

- Taste and adjust the sweetness with honey or maple syrup, if desired.
- Serve the oatmeal hot in bowls, and garnish with additional fresh fruit and almonds on top, if desired.

Cooking Tips:

- Use rolled oats instead of instant oats for a heartier texture and better nutrient content.
- Opt for mixed fresh fruits that are low in oxalate, such as berries, cherries, apples, or peaches, to help prevent kidney stone formation.
- Avoid adding nuts or seeds that are high in oxalate, such as cashews, almonds, or sesame seeds, in excessive amounts, as they may contribute to kidney stone formation.
- You can adjust the sweetness of the oatmeal by adding honey or maple syrup to your liking, but be mindful of the sugar content if you have dietary restrictions or concerns.
- If you prefer a creamier oatmeal, you can use milk or a dairy-free alternative instead of water, but be mindful of the calcium content if you have a history of calcium oxalate stones.

COCONUT MILK AND MANGO SMOOTHIE

Ingredients:

- 1 ripe mango, peeled and diced
- 1 cup coconut milk (unsweetened)
- 1/2 cup plain Greek yogurt (low-fat or non-fat)
- 1 tablespoon honey or maple syrup (optional for sweetness)
- 1/2 teaspoon fresh ginger, grated (optional)
- Ice cubes (optional for extra chill)

Cooking Instructions:

- Prepare the mango by peeling and dicing it into small pieces.
- In a blender, add the diced mango, coconut milk, Greek yogurt, honey or maple syrup (if using), and fresh ginger (if using).
- Blend all the ingredients together until smooth and creamy.
- Taste and adjust sweetness or ginger level according to your preference.
- If desired, add a few ice cubes to the blender and blend again to make the smoothie colder.
- Pour the smoothie into glasses and serve immediately.

Cooking Tips:

- Choose a ripe mango for maximum natural sweetness and flavor in the smoothie.

- You can use either fresh or frozen mango for this recipe. If using frozen mango, you may not need to add ice cubes as the smoothie will already be chilled.

- Use unsweetened coconut milk to keep the added sugars low. You can find coconut milk in the dairy or non-dairy milk section of most grocery stores.

- Greek yogurt adds creaminess and protein to the smoothie. Choose low-fat or non-fat Greek yogurt for a healthier option.

- Adjust the sweetness level with honey or maple syrup according to your taste preference, but be mindful of added sugars if you have kidney stone concerns.

- Fresh ginger adds a refreshing zing to the smoothie and is believed to have anti-inflammatory properties, which may be beneficial for kidney stone prevention. However, if you have any medical conditions or concerns, consult with a healthcare professional before adding ginger to your diet.

APPLE CINNAMON OVERNIGHT CHIA PUDDING

Ingredients:

- 1/4 cup chia seeds
- 1 cup unsweetened almond milk (or any milk of your choice)
- 1 medium apple, peeled and diced
- 1/2 teaspoon ground cinnamon
- 1/4 teaspoon vanilla extract
- 1 tablespoon honey (optional, adjust to taste)
- Chopped nuts (such as almonds or walnuts) for garnish (optional)

Instructions:

- In a medium-sized mixing bowl, whisk together chia seeds, almond milk, cinnamon, vanilla extract, and honey (if using) until well combined.
- Add in the diced apple and stir gently to distribute evenly.
- Cover the bowl with plastic wrap or a tight-fitting lid and refrigerate overnight, or for at least 4-6 hours, to allow the

chia seeds to absorb the liquid and form a pudding-like consistency.

- Before serving, give the mixture a good stir to break up any clumps and evenly distribute the ingredients.
- Serve the Apple Cinnamon Overnight Chia Pudding chilled, garnished with chopped nuts if desired.

Cooking Tips:

- Soaking the chia seeds overnight allows them to absorb the liquid and form a gel-like consistency, resulting in a creamy pudding texture.
- You can adjust the sweetness of the pudding by adding more or less honey, depending on your preference and dietary restrictions. Be mindful of your sugar intake if you have kidney stones or other health concerns.
- Feel free to customize the recipe by adding other kidney-friendly ingredients such as sliced almonds, diced pears, or ground flaxseed for added flavor and nutrition.
- If you prefer a smoother texture, you can blend the mixture in a blender or food processor before refrigerating to create a smoother pudding.

- Remember to drink plenty of water throughout the day to stay hydrated, as proper hydration is important for kidney stone prevention.

VEGGIE BREAKFAST TACOS WITH BLACK BEANS AND AVOCADO

Ingredients:

- 6 small corn tortillas
- 1 tablespoon olive oil
- 1 small red onion, diced
- 1 small bell pepper, diced
- 1 small zucchini, diced
- 1 teaspoon cumin powder
- 1/2 teaspoon smoked paprika
- 1/4 teaspoon cayenne pepper (optional)
- 1 cup cooked black beans
- Salt and pepper, to taste
- 6 large eggs
- 1 ripe avocado, diced
- Fresh cilantro, chopped, for garnish
- Lime wedges, for serving

Cooking Instructions:

- Heat a large skillet over medium heat and warm the corn tortillas for about 30 seconds on each side until they are pliable. Remove from the skillet and set aside.

- In the same skillet, add olive oil and heat over medium heat. Add the diced red onion, bell pepper, and zucchini, and sauté for 3-4 minutes until they start to soften.

- Add cumin powder, smoked paprika, and cayenne pepper (if using) to the skillet, and stir to coat the vegetables with the spices.

- Add the cooked black beans to the skillet and cook for another 2-3 minutes, stirring occasionally. Season with salt and pepper to taste.

- Create small wells in the vegetable mixture and crack one egg into each well. Cook for about 4-5 minutes until the egg whites are set but the yolks are still slightly runny.

- Carefully transfer each veggie breakfast taco with a spatula to a serving plate, making sure to keep the yolk intact.

- Top each taco with diced avocado and chopped cilantro for garnish. Serve with lime wedges on the side for an extra burst of flavor.

Cooking Tips:

- Use fresh vegetables for maximum flavor and nutrition. You can also customize the veggies to your liking, such as adding mushrooms, spinach, or tomatoes.

- If you prefer a milder spice level, you can reduce or omit the cayenne pepper.

- Make sure to season with salt and pepper to taste, but be mindful of your sodium intake if you have kidney stone illness. Consult with a healthcare professional or registered dietitian for specific dietary recommendations.

- Be careful when transferring the veggie breakfast tacos to a serving plate to avoid breaking the yolks.

- Serve with lime wedges on the side for added citrusy flavor, which can help enhance the taste of the dish.

- Enjoy these veggie breakfast tacos as part of a well-balanced diet that aligns with your individual dietary needs and restrictions, including kidney stone illness. Stay hydrated and follow a healthy eating plan recommended by your healthcare professional or registered dietitian for optimal kidney health.

CUCUMBER SALAD WITH LEMON AND DILL

Ingredients:

- 2 large cucumbers, thinly sliced
- 1/4 cup fresh lemon juice
- 2 tablespoons extra-virgin olive oil
- 1 tablespoon chopped fresh dill
- 1/2 teaspoon salt
- 1/4 teaspoon black pepper
- Optional: 1/4 red onion, thinly sliced (if tolerated)
- Optional: 1/4 cup crumbled feta cheese (if tolerated)

Instructions:

- Thinly slice the cucumbers and place them in a large mixing bowl.
- In a separate small bowl, whisk together the lemon juice, olive oil, chopped dill, salt, and black pepper to create the dressing.

- Pour the dressing over the sliced cucumbers in the mixing bowl.
- Toss the cucumbers gently with the dressing until well coated.
- If desired, add thinly sliced red onion and crumbled feta cheese (if tolerated) for extra flavor and texture.
- Let the salad marinate in the refrigerator for at least 15-30 minutes to allow the flavors to meld.
- Serve chilled as a refreshing side dish or a light salad.

Cooking Tips:

- Drink plenty of water throughout the day to stay well-hydrated, as proper hydration is crucial for kidney stone prevention.
- Limit or avoid high-oxalate foods such as spinach, beets, sweet potatoes, and nuts, as they can contribute to the formation of kidney stones in susceptible individuals.
- Use fresh lemon juice in the dressing, as lemon has been shown to have a beneficial effect in preventing kidney stones due to its citric acid content.
- Choose extra-virgin olive oil for its heart-healthy monounsaturated fats, which can be beneficial for overall health.

- Opt for low-sodium ingredients and limit added salt in the recipe, as excessive sodium intake can contribute to kidney stone formation in some cases.

GREEK HUMMUS WITH FRESH VEGETABLES

Ingredients:

- 1 can of chickpeas (15 oz), drained and rinsed
- 2 cloves of garlic, minced
- 1/4 cup of fresh lemon juice
- 1/4 cup of tahini (sesame paste)
- 2 tbsp of extra virgin olive oil
- 1 tsp of ground cumin
- 1/2 tsp of paprika
- Salt and pepper to taste
- Fresh vegetables for serving (such as cucumbers, bell peppers, carrots, cherry tomatoes, etc.)

Cooking Instructions:

- In a food processor or blender, combine the drained chickpeas, minced garlic, lemon juice, tahini, olive oil, cumin, paprika, salt, and pepper.
- Process the ingredients until smooth and creamy, scraping down the sides of the bowl as needed.
- Taste and adjust the seasoning with more salt, pepper, or lemon juice, as desired.
- Transfer the hummus to a serving bowl and refrigerate for at least 30 minutes to allow the flavors to meld.
- Wash and prepare the fresh vegetables for serving by washing, peeling, and cutting them into bite-sized pieces.
- Serve the Greek hummus with the fresh vegetables for dipping.

Cooking Tips:

- To make the hummus creamier, you can add a little more olive oil or water while blending, until you reach your desired consistency.
- If you prefer a milder garlic flavor, you can use roasted garlic or reduce the amount of minced garlic.
- You can customize the seasoning by adding other herbs and spices such as fresh parsley, oregano, or smoked paprika to suit your taste preferences.

- For kidney stone prevention, you can use low-sodium canned chickpeas and reduce the amount of added salt to control sodium intake.
- Drinking plenty of water and maintaining proper hydration is crucial for kidney stone prevention, so remember to stay well-hydrated while enjoying this hummus and vegetable dish.

ROASTED CHICKPEAS WITH HERBS AND SPICES

Ingredients:

- 1 can (15 oz) chickpeas (garbanzo beans), drained and rinsed
- 2 tbsp olive oil
- 1 tsp cumin
- 1 tsp paprika
- 1/2 tsp turmeric
- 1/2 tsp coriander
- 1/4 tsp cayenne pepper (adjust to taste)
- 1/2 tsp salt (adjust to taste)
- Freshly ground black pepper, to taste
- Fresh herbs (such as parsley, cilantro, or rosemary), chopped (optional)

Cooking Instructions:

- Preheat your oven to 400°F (200°C) and line a baking sheet with parchment paper for easy cleanup.

- In a bowl, combine the drained and rinsed chickpeas with olive oil, cumin, paprika, turmeric, coriander, cayenne pepper, salt, and black pepper. Toss well to coat the chickpeas evenly with the spices.

- Spread the seasoned chickpeas in a single layer on the prepared baking sheet.

- Roast the chickpeas in the preheated oven for 20-25 minutes, stirring occasionally, until they are crispy and golden brown.

- Remove from the oven and let the roasted chickpeas cool slightly.

- Optional: Sprinkle freshly chopped herbs (such as parsley, cilantro, or rosemary) over the roasted chickpeas for added flavor and freshness.

- Serve the roasted chickpeas as a crunchy and nutritious snack or as a topping for salads, soups, or other dishes.

Cooking Tips:

- Drink plenty of water: Staying well-hydrated is important for kidney stone prevention. Make sure to drink enough water throughout the day to help flush out toxins and prevent the formation of kidney stones.

- Limit sodium: High sodium intake can increase the risk of kidney stone formation. Be mindful of the salt content in your recipe and adjust accordingly.

- Use kidney-friendly herbs and spices: Some herbs and spices, such as parsley, cilantro, and rosemary, are believed to have potential benefits for kidney health. Consider adding them to your roasted chickpeas for added flavor and potential kidney stone prevention properties.

- Adjust spice levels: Spices like cumin, paprika, turmeric, and coriander are known for their antioxidant and anti-inflammatory properties, which may benefit kidney health. Adjust the spice levels to your taste preferences, and consult with your healthcare provider if you have any specific dietary restrictions or concerns.

- Portion control: While roasted chickpeas can be a healthy snack, they are also high in calories and carbohydrates. Practice portion control and enjoy them in moderation as part of a well-balanced diet.

FRESH FRUIT SALAD WITH MINT AND LIME

Ingredients:

- 1 cup watermelon, cubed
- 1 cup honeydew melon, cubed
- 1 cup cantaloupe, cubed
- 1 cup strawberries, halved
- 1 cup blueberries
- 2 tablespoons fresh mint leaves, chopped
- 1 tablespoon fresh lime juice
- 1 teaspoon honey (optional)

Instructions:

- Wash and prepare all the fruits. Cut the watermelon, honeydew melon, and cantaloupe into bite-sized cubes. Halve the strawberries. Rinse the blueberries.
- In a large mixing bowl, combine the watermelon, honeydew melon, cantaloupe, strawberries, and blueberries.
- In a small bowl, whisk together the fresh lime juice and honey (if using) to create the dressing.

- Pour the dressing over the fruit in the mixing bowl and gently toss to coat the fruits with the dressing.
- Add the chopped fresh mint leaves to the fruit salad and gently toss again to distribute the mint evenly.
- Refrigerate the fruit salad for at least 30 minutes to allow the flavors to meld.
- Serve chilled and enjoy!

Cooking Tips:

- Choose fresh, ripe fruits for the best flavor and nutritional value.
- Feel free to adjust the amount of honey or lime juice in the dressing to suit your taste preferences.
- You can use a variety of fruits in this salad based on your personal preferences and seasonal availability. Other kidney stone-friendly fruits include oranges, cherries, and grapes.
- Mint and lime add a refreshing flavor to the fruit salad, but you can omit them if you do not enjoy those flavors.
- To make the fruit salad ahead of time, you can prepare the fruits and dressing separately and refrigerate them. Combine them just before serving to keep the fruits fresh and prevent them from becoming too soggy.

VEGGIE SUSHI ROLLS WITH BROWN RICE AND AVOCADO

Ingredients:

- 1 cup of short-grain brown rice
- 2 cups of water
- 2 tablespoons of rice vinegar
- 1 tablespoon of sugar
- 1/2 teaspoon of salt
- 4 nori sheets (seaweed sheets)
- 1 avocado, thinly sliced
- 1 small cucumber, julienned
- 1 small carrot, julienned
- 1/2 small red bell pepper, thinly sliced
- 1/2 small yellow bell pepper, thinly sliced
- Low-sodium soy sauce, for dipping
- Pickled ginger, for serving (optional)

Cooking Instructions:

- Rinse the brown rice in cold water until the water runs clear.

- In a saucepan, combine the rinsed brown rice with 2 cups of water and bring to a boil. Reduce the heat to low, cover, and simmer for 35-40 minutes, or until the rice is cooked and tender.
- In a small bowl, mix together the rice vinegar, sugar, and salt until the sugar and salt dissolve.
- Once the rice is cooked, transfer it to a large bowl and gently fold in the rice vinegar mixture while the rice is still hot. Allow the rice to cool to room temperature.
- Place a nori sheet on a clean and dry sushi rolling mat or a flat surface.
- Spread a thin layer of brown rice evenly over the nori sheet, leaving about 1 inch of the nori sheet uncovered at the top.
- Arrange slices of avocado, cucumber, carrot, red bell pepper, and yellow bell pepper in a row across the middle of the rice.
- Using the sushi rolling mat or your fingers, tightly roll up the sushi, applying gentle pressure to hold the filling in place.
- Repeat the process with the remaining nori sheets and filling ingredients.
- Once all the rolls are assembled, use a sharp knife to slice the sushi rolls into bite-sized pieces.
- Serve the Veggie Sushi Rolls with low-sodium soy sauce for dipping and pickled ginger on the side (optional).

Cooking Tips:

- Use short-grain brown rice for the best results, as it is stickier and holds together well for sushi rolls.

- Let the rice cool to room temperature before using it for sushi rolls, as hot rice can make the nori sheets soggy.

- Use fresh and crisp veggies for the filling, such as cucumber, carrot, and bell peppers, to add crunch and texture to the sushi rolls.

- Opt for low-sodium soy sauce to reduce sodium intake, which is beneficial for kidney stone prevention.

- Drink plenty of water while consuming sushi rolls to stay hydrated, as proper hydration is essential for kidney stone prevention.

EDAMAME WITH SEA SALT

Ingredients:

- 1 cup frozen edamame
- 1 tablespoon sea salt

Instructions:

- Bring a pot of water to a boil and add a pinch of sea salt.
- Add frozen edamame to the boiling water and cook for 3-5 minutes, or until the edamame is tender but still slightly firm.
- Drain the edamame and transfer to a bowl.
- Sprinkle the sea salt over the hot edamame and toss to coat evenly.
- Serve the edamame with sea salt as a healthy and delicious snack.

Cooking Tips:

- Drink plenty of water throughout the day to stay hydrated, as proper hydration is essential for kidney stone prevention.
- Limit the amount of added salt in the recipe, as high sodium intake can increase the risk of kidney stone formation. Using sea salt sparingly can help keep the dish kidney-friendly.
- Avoid overcooking the edamame, as overcooking can cause loss of nutrients. Cook the edamame until it is tender but still slightly firm for maximum nutritional benefits.
- Feel free to customize the recipe by adding additional herbs, spices, or seasonings to suit your taste preferences, while

keeping in mind to avoid excessive use of high-sodium ingredients.

CAPRESE SALAD WITH TOMATOES, FRESH MOZZARELLA, AND BASIL

Ingredients:

- 4 ripe tomatoes, sliced
- 8 ounces fresh mozzarella cheese, sliced
- Fresh basil leaves
- Balsamic glaze (optional)
- Extra virgin olive oil
- Salt and pepper, to taste

Cooking Instructions:

- Arrange the sliced tomatoes and fresh mozzarella cheese on a serving plate, alternating between the two.
- Place fresh basil leaves on top of the tomatoes and mozzarella slices.
- Drizzle the salad with balsamic glaze (if using) and extra virgin olive oil.

- Season with a pinch of salt and a dash of pepper to taste.

Cooking Tips:

- Hydration is key: Drink plenty of water throughout the day to maintain proper hydration, which can help prevent the formation of kidney stones.
- Choose ripe tomatoes: Ripe tomatoes are typically sweeter and more flavorful, which can add depth of flavor to the salad without the need for additional salt or seasonings.
- Use fresh mozzarella: Fresh mozzarella is lower in sodium compared to processed mozzarella, which can help lower the overall sodium content of the salad.
- Be mindful of balsamic glaze: Balsamic glaze can be high in sugar and sodium, so use it sparingly or opt for a lower-sodium version.
- Use extra virgin olive oil: Extra virgin olive oil is a healthier option compared to other types of oils, as it is rich in monounsaturated fats and has anti-inflammatory properties.
- Season with herbs and spices: Fresh basil leaves are a great addition to the salad, and you can also add other herbs and spices like oregano, thyme, or garlic for added flavor without adding extra sodium.

GREEK YOGURT DIP WITH ASSORTED RAW VEGETABLES

Ingredients:

- 1 cup Greek yogurt (low-fat or non-fat)
- 1/2 cucumber, finely grated and squeezed to remove excess moisture
- 1/4 cup chopped fresh dill
- 1/4 cup chopped fresh parsley
- 1 clove garlic, minced
- 1 tbsp freshly squeezed lemon juice
- 1 tbsp extra-virgin olive oil
- Salt and pepper to taste
- Assorted raw vegetables, such as carrots, bell peppers, cucumbers, celery, and cherry tomatoes, for dipping

Cooking Instructions:

- In a medium bowl, combine the Greek yogurt, grated cucumber, dill, parsley, minced garlic, lemon juice, olive oil, salt, and pepper. Mix well to combine.

- Taste and adjust seasoning as desired with more salt, pepper, or lemon juice.
- Transfer the dip to a serving bowl and refrigerate for at least 30 minutes to allow the flavors to meld.
- Wash and prepare the assorted raw vegetables by cutting them into sticks or bite-sized pieces for dipping.
- Serve the Greek yogurt dip with the assorted raw vegetables for a healthy and refreshing snack.

Cooking Tips:

- To optimize this dip for kidney stone prevention, you can choose low-fat or non-fat Greek yogurt to reduce the intake of saturated fat, which can contribute to kidney stone formation.
- Including fresh herbs like dill and parsley in the dip adds flavor without adding extra sodium, which is beneficial for individuals who need to limit their sodium intake due to kidney stone issues.
- Grating and squeezing the cucumber helps to remove excess moisture, which can prevent the dip from becoming too watery.
- If you prefer a milder garlic flavor, you can use roasted or sautéed garlic instead of raw garlic in the dip.

- Refrigerating the dip for at least 30 minutes allows the flavors to meld and develop, resulting in a more flavorful dip.

AVOCADO AND TOMATO BRUSCHETTA

Ingredients:

- 1 ripe avocado, pitted and diced
- 1 cup cherry tomatoes, halved
- 1 clove garlic, minced
- 2 tablespoons fresh basil, finely chopped
- 2 tablespoons red onion, finely chopped
- 1 tablespoon balsamic vinegar
- 1 tablespoon extra virgin olive oil
- Salt and pepper to taste
- Whole grain baguette or bread of your choice

Cooking Instructions:

- Preheat your oven to 350°F (175°C).
- Slice the whole grain baguette or bread of your choice into thin slices and arrange them on a baking sheet. Toast the

slices in the preheated oven for about 5-7 minutes, or until they are lightly crispy. Remove from the oven and set aside.

- In a mixing bowl, combine the diced avocado, halved cherry tomatoes, minced garlic, finely chopped basil, finely chopped red onion, balsamic vinegar, and extra virgin olive oil. Season with salt and pepper to taste.
- Gently mix all the ingredients together until well combined, being careful not to mash the avocado.
- Let the avocado and tomato mixture sit for about 10 minutes to allow the flavors to meld together.
- Spoon the avocado and tomato mixture onto the toasted bread slices, spreading it evenly.
- Serve the Avocado and Tomato Bruschetta as a delicious and kidney-stone friendly appetizer or snack.

Cooking Tips:

- Choose ripe avocados for the best flavor and texture. A ripe avocado should be slightly soft when gently squeezed, but not too mushy.
- Opt for whole grain bread, such as whole grain baguette or whole wheat bread, as it is higher in fiber and may be beneficial for kidney stone prevention.

- Be mindful of portion sizes, as avocados are high in calories and should be consumed in moderation as part of a kidney-stone friendly diet.

- If desired, you can add additional kidney-stone friendly ingredients such as chopped fresh parsley, lemon juice, or diced cucumber to the avocado and tomato mixture for added flavor and nutrition.

SWEET POTATO CHIPS WITH ROSEMARY AND SEA SALT

Ingredients:

- 2 large sweet potatoes, washed and peeled
- 2 tablespoons extra-virgin olive oil
- 1 tablespoon fresh rosemary, finely chopped
- 1/2 teaspoon sea salt (or to taste)

Cooking Instructions:

- Preheat your oven to 375°F (190°C) and line a baking sheet with parchment paper.

- Slice the peeled sweet potatoes into thin, even rounds using a sharp knife or a mandolin slicer.
- In a large bowl, toss the sweet potato slices with olive oil, fresh rosemary, and sea salt, making sure each slice is coated evenly.
- Arrange the sweet potato slices in a single layer on the prepared baking sheet, making sure they do not overlap.
- Bake in the preheated oven for 12-15 minutes, or until the edges are crispy and lightly golden brown. Keep an eye on them as they can quickly over-brown.
- Remove the baking sheet from the oven and allow the chips to cool slightly before serving.

Cooking Tips:

- Choose fresh rosemary, as it is a fragrant herb that adds flavor without the need for excessive salt, which can contribute to kidney stone formation.
- Opt for extra-virgin olive oil, which is a healthier oil option that contains monounsaturated fats, known to be beneficial for heart health.
- Use sea salt sparingly or consider omitting it altogether, as excess salt intake can contribute to kidney stone formation in some cases.

- Keep the sweet potato slices thin and uniform in size to ensure they cook evenly and become crispy without burning.

- Avoid using any additional seasonings or spices that may contain high amounts of sodium or oxalate, which can be harmful for kidney stone patients.

Salad and Soup Recipes:

SPINACH AND STRAWBERRY SALAD WITH BALSAMIC VINAIGRETTE

Ingredients:

[For the salad]:

- 4 cups fresh spinach leaves, washed and dried
- 1 cup strawberries, hulled and halved
- 1/4 cup red onion, thinly sliced
- 1/4 cup crumbled feta cheese (optional)
- 1/4 cup chopped walnuts (optional)

[For the balsamic vinaigrette]:

- 2 tablespoons balsamic vinegar
- 2 tablespoons extra-virgin olive oil
- 1 teaspoon Dijon mustard
- 1 teaspoon honey
- Salt and pepper to taste

Cooking Instructions:

113 |Kidney Stone Diet Cookbook

- In a large salad bowl, combine the fresh spinach, strawberries, red onion, feta cheese (if using), and walnuts (if using).

- In a separate small bowl, whisk together the balsamic vinegar, olive oil, Dijon mustard, honey, salt, and pepper to make the balsamic vinaigrette.

- Drizzle the balsamic vinaigrette over the salad ingredients in the large bowl.

- Gently toss the salad to coat the ingredients evenly with the dressing.

- Serve immediately and enjoy!

Cooking Tips:

- Choose fresh, high-quality ingredients for the salad, including fresh spinach, ripe strawberries, and a good-quality balsamic vinegar and olive oil.

- Drink plenty of water throughout the day to stay well-hydrated, as proper hydration is important for kidney stone prevention.

- Limit the amount of added salt in the salad, as excessive salt intake can increase the risk of kidney stones. You can use herbs, spices, and other flavorings to enhance the taste of the salad without relying heavily on salt.

LENTIL AND VEGETABLE SOUP

Ingredients:

- 1 tablespoon olive oil
- 1 onion, chopped
- 2 carrots, peeled and diced
- 2 celery stalks, diced
- 3 cloves garlic, minced
- 1 teaspoon dried thyme
- 1 teaspoon dried rosemary
- 1 bay leaf
- 1 cup dried green or brown lentils, rinsed and drained
- 8 cups low-sodium vegetable broth
- 1 can (14 oz) diced tomatoes, undrained
- 2 cups chopped leafy greens (such as spinach or kale)
- Salt and pepper to taste
- Fresh parsley for garnish (optional)

Cooking Instructions:

- Heat olive oil in a large pot or Dutch oven over medium heat.

- Add chopped onion, carrots, and celery. Cook for 5-7 minutes until vegetables are softened.
- Add minced garlic, dried thyme, dried rosemary, and bay leaf. Cook for another 1-2 minutes until fragrant.
- Add lentils, vegetable broth, and diced tomatoes with their juice. Bring to a boil.
- Reduce heat to low and let the soup simmer for about 25-30 minutes until lentils are tender.
- Stir in chopped leafy greens and let them wilt for a few minutes.
- Season with salt and pepper to taste.
- Remove bay leaf before serving.
- Ladle the hot soup into bowls and garnish with fresh parsley if desired.

Cooking Tips:

- Be sure to rinse and drain the lentils before adding them to the soup. This helps remove any impurities and reduces the risk of kidney stone formation.
- Opt for low-sodium vegetable broth to keep the sodium levels in the soup in check, as high sodium intake can contribute to kidney stone formation.

- Use plenty of vegetables, such as carrots, celery, and leafy greens, which are rich in nutrients and fiber that can support kidney health.
- Avoid adding excess salt to the soup, as excessive sodium intake can increase the risk of kidney stone formation.
- Drink plenty of water and stay properly hydrated, as it is crucial for kidney stone prevention. Water helps flush out waste products from the body and dilutes urine, reducing the risk of stone formation.

GREEK SALAD WITH GRILLED CHICKEN AND LEMON DRESSING

Ingredients:

[For the Salad]:

- 1 pound of boneless, skinless chicken breast, grilled and sliced
- 4 cups of mixed greens (such as lettuce, spinach, or arugula)
- 1 small red onion, thinly sliced
- 1 cucumber, peeled and diced
- 1 cup of cherry tomatoes, halved

- 1/2 cup of kalamata olives
- 1/2 cup of crumbled feta cheese
- Fresh parsley or basil, for garnish (optional)

[For the Lemon Dressing]:

- 1/4 cup of freshly squeezed lemon juice
- 1/4 cup of extra-virgin olive oil
- 1 clove of garlic, minced
- 1 teaspoon of dried oregano
- Salt and pepper to taste

Cooking Instructions:

- Start by grilling the chicken breast until cooked through, then slice it into thin strips.
- In a large salad bowl, combine the mixed greens, sliced red onion, diced cucumber, cherry tomatoes, kalamata olives, and crumbled feta cheese.
- In a small bowl, whisk together the lemon juice, olive oil, minced garlic, dried oregano, salt, and pepper to make the lemon dressing.
- Pour the lemon dressing over the salad and toss to coat the ingredients evenly.
- Add the grilled chicken slices on top of the salad.

- Garnish with fresh parsley or basil, if desired.
- Serve the Greek Salad with Grilled Chicken and Lemon Dressing as a main dish or side dish.

Cooking Tips:

- Limit the use of added salt in the dressing and salad, as excess sodium intake can increase the risk of kidney stone formation.
- Choose low-fat or reduced-fat feta cheese to reduce saturated fat intake, as high intake of saturated fats may increase the risk of kidney stones.
- Opt for lean cuts of chicken breast for grilling, as they are lower in saturated fat compared to darker meat cuts.
- You can add more kidney stone-friendly ingredients to the salad, such as chopped fresh parsley, basil, or mint, which are known for their potential diuretic properties that may help promote urine production and flush out waste products from the kidneys.

QUINOA AND VEGGIE SALAD WITH LEMON-HERB DRESSING

Ingredients:

[For the Salad]:

- 1 cup quinoa, rinsed and drained
- 2 cups water
- 1/2 cup diced cucumber
- 1/2 cup diced bell pepper (any color)
- 1/2 cup cherry tomatoes, halved
- 1/4 cup chopped fresh parsley
- 1/4 cup chopped fresh cilantro
- 1/4 cup diced red onion
- 1/4 cup crumbled feta cheese (optional)
- Salt and pepper to taste

[For the Lemon-Herb Dressing]:

- 3 tablespoons freshly squeezed lemon juice
- 2 tablespoons extra-virgin olive oil
- 1 clove garlic, minced
- 1 teaspoon Dijon mustard
- 1 teaspoon honey or maple syrup

- 1/2 teaspoon dried oregano
- 1/2 teaspoon dried thyme
- Salt and pepper to taste

Cooking Instructions:

- In a medium saucepan, combine the quinoa and water. Bring to a boil over high heat, then reduce heat to low, cover, and simmer for about 15-20 minutes, or until the quinoa is tender and the water is absorbed. Remove from heat and let it cool to room temperature.
- In a large mixing bowl, combine the cooled quinoa, cucumber, bell pepper, cherry tomatoes, parsley, cilantro, red onion, and crumbled feta cheese (if using). Season with salt and pepper to taste.
- In a small bowl, whisk together the lemon juice, olive oil, minced garlic, Dijon mustard, honey or maple syrup, dried oregano, dried thyme, salt, and pepper to make the lemon-herb dressing.
- Pour the dressing over the quinoa and veggie mixture and toss gently to coat all the ingredients with the dressing.
- Taste and adjust seasoning if needed. You can serve the salad immediately, or refrigerate for a few hours to let the flavors meld before serving.

Cooking Tips:

- Rinse the quinoa thoroughly before cooking to remove any bitterness or saponins.
- You can use any color of bell pepper in this salad, or a combination of colors for added visual appeal.
- Feel free to customize the veggies in the salad based on your personal preferences or what you have on hand. You can add or substitute with other kidney stone-friendly veggies such as kale, spinach, zucchini, or carrots.
- If you're watching your sodium intake, you can skip adding additional salt to the salad and adjust the seasoning with herbs, lemon juice, and other low-sodium seasonings.
- To make this recipe vegan, omit the feta cheese or use a plant-based cheese alternative.

MINESTRONE SOUP WITH VEGETABLES AND BEANS

Ingredients:

- 2 tablespoons olive oil
- 1 medium onion, finely chopped

- 2 cloves garlic, minced
- 2 carrots, peeled and diced
- 2 celery stalks, diced
- 1 small zucchini, diced
- 1 cup chopped tomatoes (fresh or canned)
- 1 teaspoon dried oregano
- 1 teaspoon dried basil
- 1/2 teaspoon dried thyme
- 1 bay leaf
- 6 cups vegetable broth or low-sodium chicken broth
- 1 cup cooked kidney beans, drained and rinsed
- 1 cup cooked cannellini beans, drained and rinsed
- 1 cup chopped kale or spinach
- Salt and pepper to taste
- Grated parmesan cheese for serving (optional)

Cooking Instructions:

- In a large pot, heat the olive oil over medium heat. Add the chopped onion and minced garlic and sauté for 3-4 minutes, or until the onion is softened and translucent.

- Add the diced carrots, celery, zucchini, chopped tomatoes, dried oregano, dried basil, dried thyme, and bay leaf to the pot. Stir well to combine.

- Add the vegetable broth or low-sodium chicken broth to the pot and bring to a boil. Once boiling, reduce heat to low and let the soup simmer for about 15-20 minutes, or until the vegetables are tender.

- Add the cooked kidney beans, cannellini beans, and chopped kale or spinach to the pot. Let the soup simmer for another 5-10 minutes, or until the beans are heated through and the kale or spinach is wilted.

- Season the soup with salt and pepper to taste. Discard the bay leaf.

- Ladle the hot soup into bowls and sprinkle with grated parmesan cheese (if using) before serving.

Cooking Tips:

- You can customize the vegetables in the soup based on your personal preferences or what you have on hand. Other kidney stone-friendly veggies that you can add or substitute with include green beans, bell peppers, cauliflower, or broccoli.

- Be sure to use low-sodium vegetable broth or chicken broth to keep the soup kidney stone-friendly, as high sodium intake may contribute to kidney stone formation.
- If you prefer a thinner soup, you can add more broth or water to adjust the consistency to your liking.
- To save time, you can use canned beans instead of cooking them from scratch. Just be sure to drain and rinse them thoroughly before adding to the soup.
- Feel free to adjust the herbs and spices to suit your taste preferences. You can also add fresh herbs such as parsley or basil for added flavor.
- If you're following a vegan or plant-based diet, you can omit the parmesan cheese or use a dairy-free cheese alternative for serving.

KALE CAESAR SALAD WITH GRILLED SALMON

Ingredients:

[For the Salad]:

- 8 cups chopped kale leaves, tough stems removed

- 1 lb salmon fillets
- 1 tablespoon olive oil
- Salt and pepper to taste
- 1/4 cup freshly grated Parmesan cheese
- 1/4 cup croutons (optional)

[For the Caesar Dressing]:

- 1/2 cup plain Greek yogurt
- 1/4 cup freshly grated Parmesan cheese
- 2 tablespoons freshly squeezed lemon juice
- 2 tablespoons extra-virgin olive oil
- 2 cloves garlic, minced
- 1 teaspoon Dijon mustard
- 1/2 teaspoon Worcestershire sauce
- Salt and pepper to taste

Cooking Instructions:

- Preheat grill or stovetop grill pan over medium-high heat.
- Season the salmon fillets with olive oil, salt, and pepper. Grill the salmon fillets for about 4-5 minutes per side, or until cooked through. Remove from the grill and let it cool for a few minutes. Once cooled, flake the salmon into bite-sized pieces.

- In a large mixing bowl, combine the chopped kale leaves, grated Parmesan cheese, and croutons (if using).
- In a small bowl, whisk together the Greek yogurt, grated Parmesan cheese, lemon juice, olive oil, minced garlic, Dijon mustard, Worcestershire sauce, salt, and pepper to make the Caesar dressing.
- Pour the Caesar dressing over the kale and toss gently to coat the leaves with the dressing.
- Add the grilled salmon on top of the dressed kale salad.
- Taste and adjust seasoning if needed. You can serve the salad immediately or refrigerate for a short time to let the flavors meld before serving.

Cooking Tips:

- Massaging the kale leaves with your hands before dressing can help to soften them and make them more palatable.
- You can use any type of kale for this salad, such as curly kale or Lacinato kale (also known as Tuscan kale).
- If you prefer a milder flavor, you can blanch the kale leaves in boiling water for a few seconds and then shock them in ice water before using them in the salad.
- You can make the Caesar dressing ahead of time and store it in an airtight container in the refrigerator for up to 3 days.

- To make this recipe gluten-free, use gluten-free croutons or omit them altogether.
- Feel free to add or substitute with other kidney stone-friendly veggies such as cherry tomatoes, cucumbers, or roasted bell peppers.

SWEET POTATO AND BLACK BEAN SALAD WITH LIME VINAIGRETTE

Ingredients:

[For the Salad]:

- 2 large sweet potatoes, peeled and diced
- 1 tablespoon olive oil
- 1 teaspoon paprika
- 1/2 teaspoon cumin
- 1/2 teaspoon salt
- 1/4 teaspoon black pepper
- 1 can (15 ounces) black beans, rinsed and drained
- 1/2 cup chopped red bell pepper
- 1/2 cup chopped red onion
- 1/4 cup chopped fresh cilantro

- 1/4 cup crumbled queso fresco or feta cheese (optional)
- Salt and pepper to taste

[For the Lime Vinaigrette]:

- 3 tablespoons freshly squeezed lime juice
- 2 tablespoons extra-virgin olive oil
- 1 clove garlic, minced
- 1 teaspoon honey or maple syrup
- 1/2 teaspoon ground cumin
- Salt and pepper to taste

Cooking Instructions:

- Preheat your oven to 400°F (200°C). In a large mixing bowl, toss the diced sweet potatoes with olive oil, paprika, cumin, salt, and black pepper until evenly coated.
- Spread the seasoned sweet potatoes in a single layer on a lined baking sheet. Roast in the preheated oven for about 25-30 minutes, or until they are tender and lightly browned, stirring occasionally for even cooking.
- Remove the roasted sweet potatoes from the oven and let them cool to room temperature.
- In a large mixing bowl, combine the cooled roasted sweet potatoes, black beans, chopped red bell pepper, chopped red

onion, cilantro, and crumbled queso fresco or feta cheese (if using). Season with salt and pepper to taste.

- In a small bowl, whisk together the lime juice, olive oil, minced garlic, honey or maple syrup, ground cumin, salt, and pepper to make the lime vinaigrette.
- Pour the lime vinaigrette over the sweet potato and black bean mixture and toss gently to coat all the ingredients with the dressing.
- Taste and adjust seasoning if needed. You can serve the salad immediately, or refrigerate for a few hours to let the flavors meld before serving.

Cooking Tips:

- You can adjust the spices in the roasted sweet potatoes to your taste preferences. Add more or less paprika, cumin, salt, or black pepper to suit your liking.
- If you prefer a spicier salad, you can add a pinch of cayenne pepper or crushed red pepper flakes to the roasted sweet potatoes for a little kick.
- Feel free to customize the veggies in the salad based on your personal preferences or what you have on hand. You can add or substitute with other kidney stone-friendly veggies such as spinach, kale, bell peppers, or tomatoes.

- If you're watching your sodium intake, you can use low-sodium black beans or skip adding additional salt to the salad and adjust the seasoning with herbs, lime juice, and other low-sodium seasonings.

GAZPACHO WITH FRESH TOMATOES AND CUCUMBERS

Ingredients:

- 4 ripe tomatoes, chopped
- 1 cucumber, peeled and chopped
- 1 red bell pepper, chopped
- 1 small red onion, finely chopped
- 2 cloves garlic, minced
- 2 cups tomato juice
- 1/4 cup red wine vinegar
- 1/4 cup extra-virgin olive oil
- 1 tablespoon freshly squeezed lemon juice
- 1 teaspoon ground cumin
- 1 teaspoon salt, or to taste
- 1/2 teaspoon black pepper, or to taste
- Fresh basil or cilantro, for garnish

Cooking Instructions:

- In a blender or food processor, combine the chopped tomatoes, cucumber, red bell pepper, red onion, and minced garlic. Blend until smooth or desired consistency is reached.

- Add the tomato juice, red wine vinegar, olive oil, lemon juice, cumin, salt, and black pepper to the blender or food processor. Blend again until well combined.

- Taste and adjust seasoning as needed with salt, pepper, or additional lemon juice.

- Transfer the Gazpacho to a bowl or pitcher and refrigerate for at least 2 hours, or until chilled and flavors have melded.

- Before serving, garnish with fresh basil or cilantro.

Cooking Tips:

- Use ripe and flavorful tomatoes for the best flavor in your Gazpacho. Look for tomatoes that are firm, fragrant, and brightly colored.

- Peel the cucumber to remove the tough skin, as it can be difficult to blend and may result in a chunky texture.

- Adjust the seasoning to your taste preference. You can add more or less salt, pepper, or lemon juice depending on your preference.
- For a smoother texture, strain the Gazpacho through a fine-mesh sieve before refrigerating to remove any larger chunks.
- Chill the Gazpacho for at least 2 hours to allow the flavors to meld and the soup to become nicely chilled before serving.

BEET AND GOAT CHEESE SALAD WITH WALNUTS AND BALSAMIC GLAZE

Ingredients:

- 4 medium beets, roasted and peeled
- 4 cups mixed salad greens
- 1/2 cup crumbled goat cheese
- 1/2 cup walnuts, chopped
- 2 tablespoons balsamic glaze
- 2 tablespoons extra-virgin olive oil
- Salt and pepper, to taste

Cooking Instructions:

- Preheat your oven to 400°F (200°C). Wash the beets thoroughly and trim off the tops and roots. Wrap each beet in aluminum foil and place on a baking sheet. Roast in the oven for 45-60 minutes, or until the beets are tender when pierced with a fork. Remove from the oven and allow to cool. Once cooled, peel the beets using a paper towel to gently rub off the skin. Cut the beets into bite-sized cubes.
- In a large salad bowl, place the mixed salad greens. Add the roasted beet cubes, crumbled goat cheese, and chopped walnuts on top.
- In a small bowl, whisk together the balsamic glaze and extra-virgin olive oil to make the dressing. Drizzle the dressing over the salad.
- Season with salt and pepper to taste.
- Gently toss the salad to coat the ingredients with the dressing.
- Serve and enjoy!

Cooking Tips:

- To roast the beets, you can also wrap them in foil and place them on a baking sheet on the grill for a smoky flavor.

- You can also use pre-cooked and peeled beets for a quicker option, available in some grocery stores.
- For added crunch and flavor, you can toast the walnuts in a dry pan over medium heat for a few minutes until lightly browned before adding them to the salad.
- Adjust the amount of balsamic glaze and olive oil in the dressing to your preference for sweetness and tanginess.
- This salad can be served as a side dish or a main course. You can also add other ingredients such as fresh herbs, avocado, or grilled chicken for additional flavor and protein.

THAI CHICKEN SALAD WITH PEANUT DRESSING

Ingredients:

[For the Salad]:

- 1 pound boneless, skinless chicken breast, cooked and thinly sliced
- 4 cups mixed salad greens
- 1 cup shredded red cabbage
- 1 cup shredded carrots
- 1/2 cup chopped cilantro

- 1/4 cup chopped scallions

- 1/4 cup chopped peanuts

[For the Peanut Dressing]:

- 1/4 cup creamy peanut butter

- 2 tablespoons rice vinegar

- 2 tablespoons low-sodium soy sauce

- 2 tablespoons freshly squeezed lime juice

- 1 tablespoon honey

- 1 tablespoon minced fresh ginger

- 1 clove garlic, minced

- 2 tablespoons water, or more as needed

Cooking Instructions:

- In a large salad bowl, combine the cooked chicken breast, mixed salad greens, shredded red cabbage, shredded carrots, cilantro, scallions, and chopped peanuts.

- In a separate small bowl, whisk together the peanut butter, rice vinegar, soy sauce, lime juice, honey, minced ginger, and minced garlic until well combined.

- Add water, one tablespoon at a time, to thin the dressing to your desired consistency.

- Drizzle the peanut dressing over the salad and toss gently to coat the ingredients evenly.
- Serve immediately and enjoy!

Cooking Tips:

- You can use leftover cooked chicken breast, grilled chicken, or rotisserie chicken for this recipe to save time.
- If you prefer a milder dressing, you can adjust the amount of ginger, garlic, or lime juice to suit your taste.
- Add more water to the dressing if you prefer a thinner consistency, or less if you like it thicker.
- Feel free to customize the salad with additional veggies or toppings of your choice, such as bean sprouts, bell peppers, or chopped fresh herbs.
- To make the salad ahead of time, store the dressing separately and add it to the salad just before serving to prevent the salad from becoming soggy.

BUTTERNUT SQUASH SOUP WITH COCONUT MILK AND GINGER

Ingredients:

- 1 medium butternut squash, peeled, seeded, and diced
- 1 small onion, chopped
- 2 cloves garlic, minced
- 1 tablespoon grated fresh ginger
- 1 tablespoon coconut oil
- 4 cups low-sodium vegetable broth
- 1 cup coconut milk
- 1 teaspoon ground cumin
- 1/2 teaspoon ground cinnamon
- 1/4 teaspoon ground nutmeg
- Salt and black pepper to taste
- Fresh cilantro or parsley, for garnish

Cooking Instructions:

- Heat the coconut oil in a large pot over medium heat. Add the chopped onion and minced garlic and sauté until fragrant and softened, about 3-4 minutes.
- Add the diced butternut squash and grated ginger to the pot and cook for another 5 minutes, stirring occasionally.
- Add the vegetable broth, coconut milk, ground cumin, ground cinnamon, and ground nutmeg to the pot. Bring to a

boil, then reduce heat to low and simmer for 15-20 minutes, or until the butternut squash is soft and easily mashed with a fork.

- Remove the pot from heat and let the soup cool slightly. Use an immersion blender or a regular blender to puree the soup until smooth.
- Return the soup to the pot and place it back on the stove over low heat. Season with salt and black pepper to taste.
- Serve hot, garnished with fresh cilantro or parsley.

Cooking Tips:

- Choose a ripe butternut squash with a firm skin and no soft spots. This will ensure a sweeter and more flavorful soup.
- Use low-sodium vegetable broth to control the sodium content of the soup, as excessive sodium intake can contribute to the formation of kidney stones.
- Adjust the amount of ginger and spices to your taste preference. Ginger has anti-inflammatory properties that may help with kidney stone prevention, and the warming spices like cumin, cinnamon, and nutmeg add depth of flavor to the soup.

- Be cautious with salt, as excessive salt intake can increase the risk of kidney stone formation. Taste the soup before adding salt and use it sparingly.
- If using a regular blender, allow the soup to cool slightly before blending, and be sure to vent the blender lid to release steam.
- Store any leftovers in an airtight container in the refrigerator for up to 3 days.

MEDITERRANEAN CHICKPEA SALAD WITH FETA AND OLIVES

Ingredients:

- 2 cups cooked chickpeas (or 1 can chickpeas, drained and rinsed)
- 1/2 cup crumbled feta cheese
- 1/2 cup Kalamata olives, pitted and halved
- 1/2 cup cherry tomatoes, halved
- 1/2 cup cucumber, diced
- 1/4 cup red onion, thinly sliced
- 2 tablespoons fresh parsley, chopped
- 2 tablespoons fresh lemon juice

- 2 tablespoons extra-virgin olive oil
- 1 teaspoon dried oregano
- 1/2 teaspoon salt, or to taste
- 1/4 teaspoon black pepper, or to taste

Cooking Instructions:

- In a large mixing bowl, combine the cooked chickpeas, crumbled feta cheese, Kalamata olives, cherry tomatoes, cucumber, red onion, and fresh parsley.
- In a separate small bowl, whisk together the fresh lemon juice, olive oil, dried oregano, salt, and black pepper to make the dressing.
- Pour the dressing over the chickpea mixture in the large bowl and toss gently to coat all the ingredients with the dressing.
- Taste and adjust seasoning as needed with salt, pepper, or additional lemon juice.
- Let the Mediterranean Chickpea Salad sit at room temperature for about 10-15 minutes to allow the flavors to meld before serving.

Cooking Tips:

- Use cooked chickpeas for the best flavor and texture. You can either cook chickpeas from scratch by soaking them overnight and then boiling them until tender, or use canned chickpeas that have been drained and rinsed.

- Choose high-quality feta cheese and Kalamata olives for authentic Mediterranean flavor. Look for feta cheese that is crumbly and tangy, and Kalamata olives that are plump and briny.

- Adjust the dressing to your taste preference. You can add more or less lemon juice, olive oil, or dried oregano depending on your preference for acidity and herbiness.

- Letting the salad sit at room temperature for a short time before serving allows the flavors to meld and develop, resulting in a more delicious salad.

- Serve the Mediterranean Chickpea Salad as a side dish, a light lunch, or a healthy appetizer. It can also be a great option for meal prep as it can be made ahead of time and stored in the refrigerator for a few days

BROCCOLI AND CHEDDAR SOUP

Ingredients:

- 2 cups broccoli florets, chopped
- 1/2 cup carrots, diced
- 1/2 cup celery, diced
- 1/4 cup onion, diced
- 2 cloves garlic, minced
- 4 cups low-sodium vegetable broth
- 1 cup low-fat milk or milk alternative (such as almond milk or soy milk)
- 1 1/2 cups shredded reduced-fat cheddar cheese
- 2 tablespoons olive oil
- 1 tablespoon all-purpose flour
- 1/2 teaspoon dried thyme
- 1/2 teaspoon dried rosemary
- 1/2 teaspoon salt, or to taste
- 1/4 teaspoon black pepper, or to taste

Cooking Instructions:

- In a large pot, heat the olive oil over medium heat. Add the onion and garlic and sauté until softened and fragrant, about 3-4 minutes.

- Add the carrots, celery, dried thyme, and dried rosemary to the pot and sauté for another 3-4 minutes, until the vegetables are slightly tender.
- Stir in the flour and cook for 1-2 minutes, stirring constantly, to create a roux.
- Slowly whisk in the vegetable broth, scraping the bottom of the pot to loosen any browned bits.
- Add the broccoli to the pot and bring the mixture to a boil. Reduce the heat and simmer for 10-15 minutes, or until the vegetables are fully cooked and tender.
- Using an immersion blender or a regular blender, carefully puree the soup until smooth. If using a regular blender, allow the soup to cool slightly before blending, and be sure to vent the blender lid to prevent pressure buildup.
- Return the soup to the pot and stir in the milk and shredded cheddar cheese. Cook over low heat, stirring frequently, until the cheese is melted and the soup is heated through.
- Season with salt and black pepper to taste. Serve hot and enjoy!

Cooking Tips:

- Use low-sodium vegetable broth to control the sodium content of the soup. High sodium intake has been linked to an increased risk of kidney stones, so it's important to choose low-sodium options when possible.

- Opt for reduced-fat cheddar cheese to lower the saturated fat content of the soup. High intake of saturated fat can contribute to the formation of kidney stones, so choosing reduced-fat cheese can be a healthier option.

- Be mindful of portion sizes. While broccoli is a healthy vegetable, it is also high in oxalate, which can contribute to the formation of kidney stones in susceptible individuals. Enjoy this soup in moderation as part of a well-balanced diet.

- If you prefer a chunkier soup, you can reserve some of the cooked vegetables before blending and stir them back into the soup after blending for added texture.

- Serve the Broccoli and Cheddar Soup as a comforting and nutritious meal on its own or pair it with a side of whole grain bread or a salad for a more satisfying meal.

TUNA SALAD WITH MIXED GREENS AND LEMON-DIJON DRESSING

Ingredients:

[For the Salad]:

- 4 cups mixed salad greens
- 1 can (5 oz) chunk light tuna, drained
- 1/2 cup cherry tomatoes, halved
- 1/4 cup red onion, thinly sliced
- 1/4 cup cucumber, diced
- 1/4 cup kalamata olives, pitted
- 2 hard-boiled eggs, peeled and halved

[For the Lemon-Dijon Dressing]:

- 2 tablespoons freshly squeezed lemon juice
- 1 tablespoon Dijon mustard
- 1/4 cup extra-virgin olive oil
- 1 teaspoon honey
- Salt and black pepper to taste

Cooking Instructions:

- In a large salad bowl, arrange the mixed salad greens as the base.
- Top the greens with drained chunk light tuna, halved cherry tomatoes, thinly sliced red onion, diced cucumber, pitted kalamata olives, and halved hard-boiled eggs.

- In a small bowl, whisk together the lemon juice, Dijon mustard, olive oil, honey, salt, and black pepper to make the dressing.
- Drizzle the Lemon-Dijon Dressing over the tuna salad and toss gently to coat.
- Serve the Tuna Salad with Mixed Greens and Lemon-Dijon Dressing immediately and enjoy!

Cooking Tips:

- Choose chunk light tuna, which is generally lower in mercury compared to other types of tuna. High mercury levels in fish can be a risk factor for kidney stones, so it's important to choose lower-mercury options.
- Opt for mixed salad greens, such as spinach, arugula, and kale, which are packed with nutrients and lower in oxalate compared to other types of salad greens. Oxalate is a compound that can contribute to kidney stone formation in susceptible individuals.
- Use fresh lemon juice in the dressing, as lemon has been shown to have potential kidney stone-preventive properties due to its citric acid content.
- Be mindful of portion sizes, especially when it comes to high-protein foods like tuna and eggs. Consuming excessive

amounts of animal protein can increase the risk of kidney stones in some individuals, so it's important to enjoy them in moderation as part of a balanced diet.

- Customize the salad by adding or substituting other kidney stone-friendly ingredients, such as bell peppers, avocado, or roasted vegetables.

Main Dish Recipes:

VEGGIE BURGER WITH SWEET POTATO FRIES

Ingredients:

[For Veggie Burger]:

- 1 can of low-sodium black beans, drained and rinsed
- 1 small sweet potato, cooked and mashed
- 1/2 cup finely chopped onion
- 1/2 cup grated zucchini
- 1/2 cup grated carrots
- 1/4 cup chopped fresh cilantro
- 1/4 cup whole wheat bread crumbs
- 1 egg
- 1 tsp ground cumin
- 1/2 tsp smoked paprika
- Salt and pepper to taste
- Olive oil for cooking

[For Sweet Potato Fries]:

- 2 medium sweet potatoes, peeled and cut into fries

- 1 tbsp olive oil
- 1/2 tsp smoked paprika
- Salt and pepper to taste
- For serving (optional):
- Whole grain burger buns
- Lettuce, tomato, onion, and other desired toppings

Cooking Instructions:

- Preheat oven to 425°F (220°C) and line a baking sheet with parchment paper.
- In a large mixing bowl, combine the drained and rinsed black beans with the mashed sweet potato, chopped onion, grated zucchini, grated carrots, cilantro, bread crumbs, egg, cumin, smoked paprika, salt, and pepper. Stir well to combine.
- Form the mixture into patties of desired size, depending on how many burgers you want to make. Place the patties on the prepared baking sheet.
- In a separate bowl, toss the sweet potato fries with olive oil, smoked paprika, salt, and pepper until evenly coated. Spread them out in a single layer on the baking sheet next to the veggie burger patties.

- Bake in the preheated oven for 20-25 minutes, flipping the veggie burger patties halfway through, until they are golden brown and cooked through, and the sweet potato fries are crispy.
- Once cooked, remove from the oven and allow the veggie burger patties and sweet potato fries to cool slightly before assembling the burgers.
- Serve the veggie burger patties on whole grain buns, topped with lettuce, tomato, onion, and other desired toppings. Serve the sweet potato fries on the side.

Cooking Tips:

- Use low-sodium black beans to reduce the sodium content of the veggie burger patties, which is beneficial for kidney stone patients who need to watch their sodium intake.
- Mash the sweet potato thoroughly to ensure it mixes well with the other ingredients and helps bind the veggie burger patties together.
- Use whole wheat bread crumbs for added fiber and nutrients, and to keep the veggie burger patties kidney-friendly.
- Opt for baking instead of frying the veggie burger patties and sweet potato fries to reduce the overall fat content of the meal.

- Season the sweet potato fries with smoked paprika for added flavor without adding extra salt.
- Customize the toppings for the veggie burger according to your taste preferences and dietary restrictions.

GREEK-STYLE GRILLED LAMB CHOPS WITH MEDITERRANEAN COUSCOUS

Ingredients:

[For the lamb chops]:

- 8 lamb chops
- 2 cloves garlic, minced
- 1 tablespoon fresh rosemary, minced
- 1 tablespoon fresh oregano, minced
- 1 tablespoon fresh thyme, minced
- 2 tablespoons extra-virgin olive oil
- Salt and black pepper to taste

[For the Mediterranean couscous]:

- 1 cup couscous
- 1 cup vegetable broth
- 1 tablespoon extra-virgin olive oil

- 1 small red bell pepper, diced
- 1 small yellow bell pepper, diced
- 1/2 cup cherry tomatoes, halved
- 1/2 cup Kalamata olives, pitted and halved
- 1/4 cup fresh parsley, chopped
- Juice of 1 lemon
- Salt and black pepper to taste

Cooking instructions:

- In a bowl, combine minced garlic, rosemary, oregano, thyme, olive oil, salt, and black pepper. Mix well to create a marinade.
- Place the lamb chops in a shallow dish and coat them with the marinade. Let them marinate for at least 30 minutes, or overnight in the refrigerator for best results.
- Preheat a grill or stovetop grill pan over medium-high heat.
- Remove the lamb chops from the marinade and grill them for about 3-4 minutes per side for medium-rare, or until desired doneness is reached. Let them rest for a few minutes before serving.
- Meanwhile, prepare the Mediterranean couscous. In a saucepan, bring the vegetable broth to a boil. Stir in the

couscous and olive oil, then cover and remove from heat. Let it sit for 5 minutes until the couscous is fluffy.

- Fluff the cooked couscous with a fork and transfer it to a large serving bowl.
- Add the diced bell peppers, halved cherry tomatoes, pitted and halved Kalamata olives, chopped parsley, lemon juice, salt, and black pepper to the couscous. Toss gently to combine.
- Serve the grilled lamb chops over the Mediterranean couscous, garnished with additional fresh herbs, if desired.

Cooking tips:

- For best results, marinate the lamb chops for at least 30 minutes, or overnight in the refrigerator. This will allow the flavors to penetrate the meat and make it more tender and flavorful.
- Make sure to rest the grilled lamb chops for a few minutes before serving. This will help the juices redistribute and result in juicier, more tender meat.
- Adjust the grilling time for the lamb chops based on your preferred level of doneness. Cooking time may vary depending on the thickness of the lamb chops and the heat of your grill or grill pan.

- You can customize the Mediterranean couscous by adding or substituting other Mediterranean ingredients such as chopped cucumber, crumbled feta cheese, or diced red onion for added flavor and nutrition.
- Stay hydrated and drink plenty of water, as it can help prevent the formation of kidney stones. Be sure to follow any dietary restrictions or recommendations provided by your healthcare provider if you have kidney stone illness or other health conditions.

TOFU AND VEGETABLE CURRY WITH BROWN RICE

Ingredients:

[For the tofu and vegetable curry]:

- 14 oz firm tofu, drained and cubed
- 1 tablespoon coconut oil
- 1 small onion, diced
- 3 cloves garlic, minced
- 1 tablespoon fresh ginger, grated
- 2 teaspoons curry powder
- 1/2 teaspoon turmeric

- 1/4 teaspoon cumin
- 1/4 teaspoon paprika
- 1/4 teaspoon red pepper flakes (optional)
- 1 small head cauliflower, cut into florets
- 2 small carrots, peeled and sliced
- 1 small zucchini, sliced
- 1 small red bell pepper, diced
- 1 can (14 oz) coconut milk
- 1 tablespoon tomato paste
- Salt and black pepper to taste
- Fresh cilantro or parsley for garnish (optional)

[For the brown rice]:

- 1 cup brown rice
- 2 cups water
- 1/2 teaspoon salt

Cooking instructions:

- Prepare the brown rice by rinsing it under cold water in a fine-mesh strainer. In a medium saucepan, combine the brown rice, water, and salt. Bring to a boil, then reduce heat to low, cover, and simmer for about 40-45 minutes, or until the rice is tender and cooked through. Fluff with a fork and set aside.

- In a large pan or wok, heat the coconut oil over medium heat. Add the diced onion and cook for 2-3 minutes until softened.
- Add the minced garlic, grated ginger, curry powder, turmeric, cumin, paprika, and red pepper flakes (if using) to the pan. Stir-fry for 1-2 minutes until fragrant.
- Add the cubed tofu to the pan and cook for 3-4 minutes until lightly browned on all sides.
- Add the cauliflower florets, sliced carrots, sliced zucchini, and diced red bell pepper to the pan. Stir-fry for 3-4 minutes until the vegetables are slightly tender.
- Stir in the coconut milk and tomato paste. Bring the mixture to a simmer and let it cook for another 5-7 minutes, stirring occasionally, until the vegetables are cooked to your desired level of tenderness and the flavors have melded together.
- Season the curry with salt and black pepper to taste.
- Serve the tofu and vegetable curry over the cooked brown rice, garnished with fresh cilantro or parsley (if desired).

Cooking tips:

- Use firm tofu for this recipe, as it holds its shape better during cooking. You can press the tofu to remove excess water for better texture and flavor.

- Adjust the curry powder and red pepper flakes to your preferred level of spiciness. You can also add more or less coconut milk to adjust the consistency of the curry sauce.

- Feel free to customize the vegetable selection based on your preferences or what's available. Other vegetables that work well in this curry include broccoli, green beans, spinach, or peas.

- Be mindful of your salt intake if you have kidney stone illness or other health conditions. You can reduce or omit salt from the recipe and use other herbs and spices to add flavor.

- Stay hydrated and drink plenty of water, as it can help prevent the formation of kidney stones. Be sure to follow any dietary restrictions or recommendations provided by your healthcare provider if you have kidney stone illness or other health conditions.

BAKED COD WITH HERBS AND TOMATOES

Ingredients:

- 4 cod fillets, about 6 ounces each
- 1 tablespoon extra-virgin olive oil
- 2 cloves garlic, minced
- 1 tablespoon fresh thyme, minced
- 1 tablespoon fresh rosemary, minced
- 1 tablespoon fresh parsley, chopped
- 1 cup cherry tomatoes, halved
- Salt and black pepper to taste
- Lemon wedges for serving

Cooking instructions:

- Preheat your oven to 375°F (190°C) and line a baking dish with parchment paper or foil for easy cleanup.
- Pat dry the cod fillets with paper towels and place them in the prepared baking dish.
- In a small bowl, mix together the olive oil, minced garlic, minced thyme, minced rosemary, chopped parsley, salt, and black pepper to create a herb mixture.
- Rub the herb mixture evenly over the top of each cod fillet, covering them well.

- Scatter the cherry tomato halves around the cod fillets in the baking dish.

- Bake in the preheated oven for 15-18 minutes, or until the cod fillets are opaque and flake easily with a fork.

- Remove from the oven and let the cod fillets rest for a few minutes before serving.

- Serve the baked cod fillets with herbs and tomatoes hot, garnished with additional chopped parsley and lemon wedges for squeezing over the top.

Cooking tips:

- Use fresh herbs for the best flavor. You can adjust the amount of herbs to your taste preferences or substitute with other fresh herbs such as basil or dill.

- Choose fresh, high-quality cod fillets for the best results. Look for fillets that are firm, moist, and have a mild, slightly sweet smell.

- If you prefer, you can use other types of white fish fillets such as haddock, halibut, or sea bass in place of cod.

- Be careful not to overcook the cod fillets as they can become dry and tough. Keep a close eye on them while baking and adjust the cooking time as needed based on the thickness of the fillets.

- Tomatoes add natural acidity and flavor to the dish, but if you have specific dietary restrictions or recommendations related to kidney stone illness, you can reduce or omit the tomatoes.

LENTIL AND VEGETABLE STIR-FRY WITH GINGER AND SOY SAUCE

Ingredients:

- 1 cup dried lentils, rinsed and drained
- 2 cups vegetable broth
- 2 tablespoons vegetable oil
- 1 tablespoon freshly grated ginger
- 3 cloves garlic, minced
- 1 small onion, thinly sliced
- 1 small carrot, julienned
- 1 small bell pepper, thinly sliced
- 1 cup broccoli florets
- 1/2 cup snow peas
- 2 tablespoons soy sauce

- 1 tablespoon rice vinegar
- 1 tablespoon sesame oil
- Salt and black pepper to taste
- Chopped green onions and sesame seeds for garnish (optional)

Cooking instructions:

- In a medium saucepan, bring the vegetable broth to a boil. Add the lentils and reduce heat to low. Simmer for about 15-20 minutes, or until the lentils are tender but not mushy. Drain any excess liquid and set aside.
- In a large wok or skillet, heat the vegetable oil over medium-high heat.
- Add the grated ginger and minced garlic to the hot oil, and sauté for about 30 seconds until fragrant.
- Add the sliced onion, julienned carrot, and bell pepper to the wok or skillet. Stir-fry for about 2-3 minutes until the vegetables start to soften.
- Add the broccoli florets and snow peas to the wok or skillet, and stir-fry for another 2-3 minutes until the vegetables are crisp-tender.
- Add the cooked lentils to the wok or skillet, and toss everything together.

- In a small bowl, whisk together soy sauce, rice vinegar, and sesame oil. Pour the sauce over the stir-fry and toss to coat evenly.
- Season with salt and black pepper to taste.
- Remove from heat and garnish with chopped green onions and sesame seeds, if desired.
- Serve the Lentil and Vegetable Stir-Fry with Ginger and Soy Sauce over cooked brown rice or quinoa for a complete meal.

Cooking tips:

- To optimize this recipe for kidney stone illness, make sure to drink plenty of water and stay hydrated to help flush out toxins and prevent the formation of kidney stones. Be sure to follow any dietary restrictions or recommendations provided by your healthcare provider.
- You can customize this stir-fry by adding or substituting other vegetables such as mushrooms, zucchini, or cauliflower based on your preference or availability.
- Adjust the cooking time for the vegetables based on your desired level of crunchiness. Stir-frying quickly over high heat helps to retain the nutrients and crispness of the vegetables.

- If you prefer a spicier stir-fry, you can add red pepper flakes or sriracha sauce to the sauce mixture for some heat.
- Leftovers can be stored in an airtight container in the refrigerator for up to 3-4 days. Reheat in a pan or microwave before serving, and add additional sauce or seasoning if needed.

GRILLED PORTOBELLO MUSHROOMS WITH BALSAMIC GLAZE

Ingredients:

- 4 large portobello mushrooms, stems removed
- 1/4 cup balsamic vinegar
- 2 tablespoons extra-virgin olive oil
- 2 cloves garlic, minced
- 1 tablespoon fresh thyme leaves
- Salt and black pepper to taste
- Fresh parsley for garnish (optional)

Cooking instructions:

- In a bowl, whisk together balsamic vinegar, olive oil, minced garlic, fresh thyme leaves, salt, and black pepper to create a marinade.
- Place the cleaned portobello mushrooms in a shallow dish and pour the marinade over them. Use a brush to coat the mushrooms evenly with the marinade.
- Let the mushrooms marinate for at least 30 minutes, or longer in the refrigerator for more intense flavor.
- Preheat a grill or stovetop grill pan over medium-high heat.
- Remove the mushrooms from the marinade and place them on the grill, gill side down. Reserve the marinade for later use.
- Grill the mushrooms for about 4-5 minutes per side, or until they are tender and grill marks appear.
- While grilling, brush the reserved marinade over the mushrooms to baste them and enhance the flavor.
- Remove the mushrooms from the grill and let them rest for a few minutes.
- Serve the grilled portobello mushrooms hot, garnished with fresh parsley, if desired.

Cooking tips:

- Make sure to clean the portobello mushrooms properly by gently wiping them with a damp cloth or paper towel to remove any dirt or debris. Avoid soaking them in water as they can absorb excess moisture and become soggy.

- Allow the mushrooms to marinate for at least 30 minutes, or longer for a more intense flavor. This will help infuse the mushrooms with the flavors of the marinade.

- Be careful not to overcook the mushrooms, as they can become mushy and lose their texture. Grill them until they are tender with grill marks, but still firm.

- You can use a basting brush to brush the reserved marinade over the mushrooms while grilling to enhance their flavor and keep them moist.

- Feel free to customize the marinade by adding other herbs or spices that you enjoy, such as rosemary, thyme, or red pepper flakes, to suit your taste preferences.

LEMON-ROSEMARY ROASTED TURKEY BREAST WITH ROASTED VEGETABLES

Ingredients:

[For the Lemon-Rosemary Roasted Turkey Breast]:

- 1 bone-in turkey breast, about 4-5 lbs
- 1/4 cup freshly squeezed lemon juice
- Zest of 1 lemon
- 2 tablespoons extra-virgin olive oil
- 2 cloves garlic, minced
- 1 tablespoon fresh rosemary leaves, finely chopped
- Salt and black pepper to taste

[For the Roasted Vegetables]:

- 4 cups mixed vegetables of your choice (such as carrots, bell peppers, zucchini, and red onions), cut into bite-sized pieces
- 2 tablespoons extra-virgin olive oil
- 1 tablespoon fresh rosemary leaves, finely chopped
- Salt and black pepper to taste

Cooking instructions:

- Preheat your oven to 375°F (190°C).
- Rinse and pat dry the turkey breast with paper towels.
- In a small bowl, whisk together lemon juice, lemon zest, olive oil, minced garlic, fresh rosemary, salt, and black pepper to create a marinade.

- Place the turkey breast in a roasting pan and pour the marinade over it. Use your hands or a brush to coat the turkey breast evenly with the marinade.

- Roast the turkey breast in the preheated oven for about 1.5 to 2 hours, or until a meat thermometer inserted into the thickest part of the breast reads 165°F (75°C).

- While the turkey breast is roasting, prepare the roasted vegetables. In a large mixing bowl, toss the mixed vegetables with olive oil, fresh rosemary, salt, and black pepper.

- Spread the vegetables in a single layer on a baking sheet lined with parchment paper.

- After the turkey breast has roasted for about 30 minutes, place the baking sheet with the vegetables in the oven and roast for about 30-40 minutes, or until the vegetables are tender and lightly browned.

- Once the turkey breast is cooked, remove it from the oven and let it rest for about 10-15 minutes before carving.

- Carve the turkey breast into slices and serve it with the roasted vegetables on the side.

Cooking tips:

- Choose a bone-in turkey breast for maximum flavor and juiciness. Bone-in turkey breasts tend to be more flavorful and moist compared to boneless ones.

- Make sure to properly rinse and pat dry the turkey breast before marinating to ensure the marinade adheres well to the meat.

- Use fresh lemon juice and zest for the marinade to add bright citrusy flavors to the turkey breast.

- Fresh rosemary is a fragrant herb that pairs well with turkey. If you don't have fresh rosemary, you can use dried rosemary, but reduce the amount by half as dried herbs are more potent.

- You can customize the roasted vegetables by using your favorite mix of vegetables. Choose a variety of colorful vegetables to add flavor, texture, and nutrition to the dish.

- Be sure to monitor the internal temperature of the turkey breast using a meat thermometer to ensure it reaches 165°F (75°C) for safe consumption.

SPAGHETTI SQUASH WITH TOMATO SAUCE AND TURKEY MEATBALLS

Ingredients:

[For the Turkey Meatballs]:

- 1 pound ground turkey
- 1/4 cup grated Parmesan cheese
- 1/4 cup breadcrumbs (use whole grain for added fiber)
- 1/4 cup chopped fresh parsley
- 1 large egg
- 2 cloves garlic, minced
- 1/2 teaspoon salt
- 1/4 teaspoon black pepper

[For the Tomato Sauce]:

- 1 tablespoon olive oil
- 1 small onion, finely chopped
- 3 cloves garlic, minced
- 1 can (28 ounces) crushed tomatoes (preferably low-sodium)
- 1 teaspoon dried oregano
- 1 teaspoon dried basil
- 1/2 teaspoon salt
- 1/4 teaspoon black pepper

[For the Spaghetti Squash]:

- 1 medium spaghetti squash

- Olive oil, for brushing
- Salt and black pepper, to taste

Cooking instructions:

- Preheat the oven to 375°F (190°C). Line a baking sheet with parchment paper.
- In a large mixing bowl, combine ground turkey, grated Parmesan cheese, breadcrumbs, chopped parsley, minced garlic, egg, salt, and black pepper. Mix well with your hands.
- Roll the mixture into small meatballs, about 1 inch in diameter.
- Place the meatballs on the prepared baking sheet and bake in the preheated oven for 15-18 minutes, or until cooked through and lightly browned. Set aside.
- In the meantime, prepare the tomato sauce. In a saucepan, heat olive oil over medium heat. Add the chopped onion and minced garlic, and sauté until softened, about 5 minutes.
- Add the crushed tomatoes, dried oregano, dried basil, salt, and black pepper to the saucepan. Bring to a simmer and let it cook for about 15 minutes, stirring occasionally.
- While the sauce is simmering, prepare the spaghetti squash. Cut the spaghetti squash in half lengthwise and scoop out the seeds with a spoon.

- Brush the cut sides of the spaghetti squash with olive oil and season with salt and black pepper.

- Place the spaghetti squash halves cut side down on a baking sheet lined with parchment paper. Bake in the preheated oven for 30-40 minutes, or until the flesh is tender and easily shreds into spaghetti-like strands with a fork.

- Once the spaghetti squash is cooked, use a fork to scrape the flesh into spaghetti-like strands.

- To serve, place a generous scoop of spaghetti squash on a plate or bowl. Top with a ladle of tomato sauce and several turkey meatballs. Garnish with additional chopped parsley, if desired.

Cooking tips:

- Drink plenty of water and stay well-hydrated, as it can help prevent kidney stones. Water is important for kidney health and can help flush out toxins and waste products from the body.

- Choose low-sodium crushed tomatoes or tomato sauce to reduce sodium intake, as high sodium intake can contribute to kidney stone formation in some cases.

- Use whole grain breadcrumbs for the turkey meatballs to increase the fiber content of the dish, which can be beneficial for kidney health.

- Be mindful of portion sizes, as overeating certain foods, including high-protein foods like meatballs, may increase the risk of kidney stones in some cases. Follow any dietary recommendations or restrictions provided by your healthcare provider.

- Feel free to customize the tomato sauce by adding other herbs or spices that you enjoy, such as fresh basil or thyme, to suit your taste preferences.

- If you're watching your salt intake, you can further reduce the sodium content by using a no-salt-added or low-sodium canned tomato product or making your own tomato sauce from fresh tomatoes.

- Choose lean ground turkey for the meatballs, as it is lower in fat compared to other types of ground meat. High-fat diets can increase the risk of kidney stone formation.

- Be sure to thoroughly cook the turkey meatballs to an internal temperature of 165°F (74°C) to ensure they are safe to eat.

- Spaghetti squash is a good source of fiber and can be a healthier alternative to traditional pasta for those with kidney stone concerns. However, moderation is key, as it still contains carbohydrates that can impact blood sugar levels. Consult with your healthcare provider or a registered dietitian for personalized dietary recommendations.

- Consider adding some kidney-friendly vegetables such as chopped spinach or zucchini to the tomato sauce for added nutrients and flavor.

- If you prefer a vegetarian option, you can omit the turkey meatballs and use plant-based protein options such as lentil or chickpea meatballs instead.

TERIYAKI CHICKEN WITH STEAMED VEGETABLES AND BROWN RICE

Ingredients:

- 4 boneless, skinless chicken breasts
- 1/2 cup low-sodium soy sauce
- 1/4 cup brown sugar
- 1/4 cup rice vinegar
- 2 tablespoons mirin (Japanese sweet rice wine)
- 2 cloves garlic, minced
- 1 tablespoon minced ginger
- 1 tablespoon cornstarch

- 2 cups mixed vegetables (such as broccoli, carrots, bell peppers)
- 2 cups cooked brown rice

Cooking Instructions:

- In a small saucepan, whisk together the soy sauce, brown sugar, rice vinegar, mirin, minced garlic, minced ginger, and cornstarch. Bring to a boil over medium heat, then reduce heat to low and simmer for 5 minutes, stirring occasionally. Remove from heat and let cool.
- Place the chicken breasts in a shallow dish and pour half of the teriyaki sauce over them, reserving the other half for later. Let the chicken marinate for 15-30 minutes.
- Preheat a grill or stovetop grill pan over medium-high heat. Grill the chicken breasts for 5-6 minutes per side or until cooked through, basting with the marinade occasionally. Remove from heat and let rest for a few minutes before slicing into strips.
- Meanwhile, steam the mixed vegetables until tender-crisp, about 5 minutes.
- To serve, divide the cooked brown rice among four plates or bowls. Top with the teriyaki chicken strips and steamed

vegetables. Drizzle with the reserved teriyaki sauce. Serve hot and enjoy!

Cooking Tips:

- Use low-sodium soy sauce to reduce the sodium content of the dish, as high sodium intake can increase the risk of kidney stone formation.

- Brown sugar can be substituted with a sugar substitute or reduced to lower the overall sugar content of the teriyaki sauce, especially if you have concerns about blood sugar levels.

- Be sure to cook the chicken breasts thoroughly to an internal temperature of 165°F (74°C) to ensure they are safe to eat.

- Choose a variety of colorful mixed vegetables for added nutrients and fiber. Avoid high-oxalate vegetables such as spinach or beets if you have a history of calcium oxalate kidney stones.

- Opt for cooked brown rice instead of white rice, as it is higher in fiber and nutrients, and can be a healthier option for kidney stone prevention.

BLACK BEAN AND SWEET POTATO ENCHILADAS WITH AVOCADO CREAM SAUCE

Ingredients:

[For the Enchiladas]:

- 8 small corn tortillas
- 1 can black beans, rinsed and drained
- 2 medium sweet potatoes, peeled and diced
- 1/2 red onion, finely chopped
- 1 clove garlic, minced
- 1 teaspoon ground cumin
- 1 teaspoon smoked paprika
- Salt and pepper to taste
- 1 tablespoon olive oil
- 1/2 cup shredded low-fat cheese (such as Monterey Jack or Cheddar), optional

[For the Avocado Cream Sauce]:

- 1 ripe avocado
- 1/4 cup plain Greek yogurt
- 1 tablespoon lime juice
- 1 clove garlic, minced

- Salt and pepper to taste

[For Garnish]:

- Chopped fresh cilantro
- Sliced jalapenos, optional

Cooking Instructions:

- Preheat your oven to 375°F (190°C). Grease a 9x13 inch baking dish and set aside.
- In a large skillet, heat the olive oil over medium heat. Add the chopped red onion and minced garlic, and sauté until softened, about 2-3 minutes.
- Add the diced sweet potatoes, ground cumin, smoked paprika, salt, and pepper to the skillet. Stir well to coat the sweet potatoes in the spices. Cook for 5-7 minutes, stirring occasionally, until the sweet potatoes are tender.
- Add the rinsed and drained black beans to the skillet, and cook for an additional 2-3 minutes to heat through. Remove from heat.
- In a separate bowl, mash the avocado until smooth. Add the Greek yogurt, lime juice, minced garlic, salt, and pepper. Stir well to combine, creating the avocado cream sauce.

- To assemble the enchiladas, warm the corn tortillas in a dry skillet or microwave for a few seconds to soften them. Place a spoonful of the black bean and sweet potato mixture onto each tortilla, and roll tightly. Place the rolled enchiladas seam-side down in the greased baking dish.
- Once all the enchiladas are assembled, pour the avocado cream sauce over the top, spreading it out evenly. If desired, sprinkle shredded cheese on top.
- Bake the enchiladas in the preheated oven for 20-25 minutes, or until the cheese is melted and bubbly (if using) and the enchiladas are heated through.
- Remove from the oven and let cool for a few minutes. Garnish with chopped fresh cilantro and sliced jalapenos, if desired, before serving.

Cooking Tips:

- Use low-sodium black beans or rinse canned black beans thoroughly to reduce sodium content, as high sodium intake can increase the risk of kidney stone formation.
- Adjust the spices to your preference. You can add more or less cumin and smoked paprika depending on your taste buds.

- Consider using whole-grain corn tortillas for added fiber and nutrients.

- Use low-fat cheese or skip the cheese altogether to reduce saturated fat and cholesterol intake, as high intake of these nutrients can be associated with an increased risk of kidney stones.

- If you prefer a spicier dish, you can add diced jalapenos or other hot peppers to the sweet potato and black bean mixture.

STEAMED BROCCOLI WITH GARLIC AND OLIVE OIL

Ingredients:

- 1 head of broccoli, washed and trimmed into florets
- 2 cloves garlic, minced
- 2 tablespoons extra virgin olive oil
- Salt and pepper to taste
- Lemon wedges, for serving (optional)

Cooking Instructions:

- Fill a large pot or steamer basket with about 1 inch of water and bring it to a boil over high heat.
- Place the broccoli florets in the steamer basket and cover with a lid. Steam the broccoli for 4-5 minutes, or until it is tender but still crisp.
- In a small saucepan, heat the olive oil over medium-low heat. Add the minced garlic and cook for 1-2 minutes, or until fragrant, being careful not to let it burn.

- Remove the steamed broccoli from the steamer basket and transfer to a serving dish.
- Drizzle the garlic-infused olive oil over the steamed broccoli. Season with salt and pepper to taste.
- Toss gently to coat the broccoli evenly with the garlic and olive oil.
- Serve hot with lemon wedges, if desired, for an extra burst of flavor.

Cooking Tips:

- Avoid overcooking the broccoli as it can result in a loss of nutrients and a mushy texture. Steaming for 4-5 minutes should leave the broccoli tender yet still crisp.
- Be cautious not to burn the minced garlic when heating the olive oil. Garlic can quickly turn bitter when overcooked.
- Use extra virgin olive oil for its heart-healthy properties and rich flavor. If desired, you can also use garlic-infused olive oil for an extra boost of garlic flavor.
- Season the broccoli with salt and pepper to taste, but be mindful of your sodium intake, especially if you are prone to kidney stones. Opt for reduced-sodium options or use herbs and spices to add flavor without excess salt.

- Squeezing fresh lemon juice over the steamed broccoli before serving can add a tangy twist and increase the dish's vitamin C content.

CILANTRO-LIME BROWN RICE

Ingredients:

- 1 cup brown rice
- 2 cups water
- 1/4 cup fresh cilantro, chopped
- 2 tablespoons freshly squeezed lime juice
- 1 tablespoon olive oil
- 1/2 teaspoon salt
- 1/4 teaspoon black pepper

Cooking Instructions:

- In a medium saucepan, combine the brown rice and water. Bring to a boil over high heat.
- Once boiling, reduce the heat to low, cover the saucepan with a lid, and simmer for about 35-40 minutes, or until the rice is cooked and tender.

- Remove the saucepan from heat and let the rice stand, covered, for 5 minutes.

- In a small bowl, whisk together the lime juice, olive oil, salt, and black pepper to make the dressing.

- Fluff the cooked rice with a fork, and then stir in the chopped cilantro.

- Pour the lime dressing over the rice, and stir gently to evenly coat the rice with the dressing.

- Taste and adjust salt and pepper as needed.

- Serve the cilantro-lime brown rice as a side dish or as a base for other Mediterranean or Mexican-inspired dishes.

Cooking Tips:

- Use low-sodium vegetable broth or water to cook the brown rice to reduce sodium intake, as high sodium intake can increase the risk of kidney stone formation.

- Rinse the brown rice thoroughly before cooking to remove excess starch and improve texture.

- You can adjust the amount of cilantro and lime juice to your preference. If you're not a fan of cilantro, you can substitute it with parsley or other fresh herbs.

- For a more pronounced citrus flavor, you can increase the amount of lime juice or add some lime zest.

- Consider using extra-virgin olive oil for its heart-healthy properties, as it contains beneficial monounsaturated fats.
- Store leftovers in an airtight container in the refrigerator for up to 3-4 days. Reheat before serving, and add a little extra lime juice and cilantro if desired to refresh the flavors.

BALSAMIC-GLAZED ROASTED CAULIFLOWER

Ingredients:

- 1 head of cauliflower, washed and cut into florets
- 3 tablespoons balsamic vinegar
- 2 tablespoons olive oil
- 2 cloves garlic, minced
- 1/2 teaspoon salt
- 1/4 teaspoon black pepper
- Fresh parsley, chopped (optional, for garnish)

Cooking Instructions:

- Preheat your oven to 400°F (200°C) and line a baking sheet with parchment paper.

- In a small bowl, whisk together the balsamic vinegar, olive oil, minced garlic, salt, and black pepper to make the glaze.
- Place the cauliflower florets in a large mixing bowl and drizzle the balsamic glaze over them. Toss to coat the cauliflower evenly.
- Arrange the coated cauliflower florets in a single layer on the prepared baking sheet.
- Roast in the preheated oven for 20-25 minutes, or until the cauliflower is tender and golden brown, stirring occasionally for even cooking.
- Remove from the oven and let cool for a few minutes.
- Garnish with chopped fresh parsley, if desired, before serving.

Cooking Tips:

- Use low-sodium balsamic vinegar and olive oil to reduce sodium intake, as high sodium intake can increase the risk of kidney stone formation.
- You can adjust the amount of balsamic vinegar and olive oil to your preference. If you prefer a sweeter glaze, you can add a little honey or maple syrup.
- Make sure to coat the cauliflower florets evenly with the glaze for maximum flavor.

- If you like a little heat, you can add a pinch of red pepper flakes or a dash of hot sauce to the glaze for a spicy kick.
- You can also add other herbs or spices to the glaze, such as rosemary, thyme, or paprika, to customize the flavor to your liking.
- Serve the Balsamic-Glazed Roasted Cauliflower as a delicious and healthy side dish or as a topping for salads, grain bowls, or roasted vegetable medleys.

GREEK-STYLE ROASTED POTATOES WITH LEMON AND OREGANO

Ingredients:

- 4 medium potatoes, peeled and cut into chunks
- 3 tablespoons olive oil
- 2 tablespoons freshly squeezed lemon juice
- 2 teaspoons dried oregano
- 1/2 teaspoon salt
- 1/4 teaspoon black pepper
- Fresh parsley, chopped (optional)

Cooking Instructions:

- Preheat your oven to 425°F (220°C) and line a baking sheet with parchment paper.
- In a large mixing bowl, combine the olive oil, lemon juice, dried oregano, salt, and black pepper. Whisk together to make the marinade.
- Add the potato chunks to the bowl with the marinade and toss to coat the potatoes evenly.
- Arrange the marinated potato chunks in a single layer on the prepared baking sheet.
- Roast the potatoes in the preheated oven for about 30-35 minutes, or until they are golden and crispy on the outside and tender on the inside, flipping them halfway through cooking for even browning.
- Remove the roasted potatoes from the oven and let them cool for a few minutes.
- Sprinkle with fresh chopped parsley, if desired, before serving.

Cooking Tips:

- You can use any type of potatoes for this recipe, such as russet, Yukon gold, or red potatoes.

- For a lower-fat option, you can reduce the amount of olive oil or use a cooking spray to coat the potatoes.
- Adjust the amount of lemon juice, oregano, salt, and pepper to your preference. You can also add additional herbs and spices, such as garlic powder or paprika, for more flavor.
- To ensure even cooking and browning, make sure to spread the potato chunks in a single layer on the baking sheet without overcrowding them.
- For a crispier texture, you can increase the oven temperature or broil the potatoes for the last few minutes of cooking.
- Leftovers can be stored in an airtight container in the refrigerator for up to 2-3 days. Reheat in the oven or on a stovetop pan for best results.

GARLIC-SAUTEED SPINACH

Ingredients:

- 1 pound fresh spinach, washed and drained
- 2 tablespoons olive oil
- 4 cloves garlic, minced
- 1/4 teaspoon red pepper flakes (optional)
- Salt and pepper to taste

Cooking Instructions:

- Heat the olive oil in a large skillet over medium heat.
- Add the minced garlic and red pepper flakes (if using) to the skillet, and sauté for 1-2 minutes until fragrant, being careful not to burn the garlic.
- Add the fresh spinach to the skillet, and toss gently to coat it with the garlic-infused oil.
- Cook the spinach for 2-3 minutes, stirring occasionally, until it wilts down and becomes tender.
- Season the spinach with salt and pepper to taste, and continue to cook for another minute or two.
- Remove the skillet from heat, and serve the garlic-sauteed spinach hot as a side dish or as a base for other Mediterranean-inspired dishes.

Cooking Tips:

- Use fresh spinach for the best flavor and nutrition. If using frozen spinach, make sure to thaw and drain it well before cooking, and adjust cooking time accordingly.
- Avoid overcooking the spinach to retain its vibrant green color and prevent nutrient loss.

- You can adjust the amount of garlic and red pepper flakes to your preference. If you're not a fan of spicy flavors, you can skip the red pepper flakes.
- Consider using extra-virgin olive oil for its heart-healthy properties, as it contains beneficial monounsaturated fats.
- Be cautious with salt intake, as high sodium intake can increase the risk of kidney stone formation. Use salt sparingly and taste as you go.
- Feel free to add other herbs or seasonings, such as lemon zest or chopped fresh herbs like parsley or basil, to enhance the flavor of the garlic-sauteed spinach.
- Store leftovers in an airtight container in the refrigerator for up to 2-3 days. Reheat before serving, and adjust seasoning as needed.

ROASTED BUTTERNUT SQUASH WITH CINNAMON AND MAPLE SYRUP

Ingredients:

- 1 medium butternut squash, peeled, seeded, and cut into 1-inch cubes
- 2 tablespoons olive oil

- 2 tablespoons pure maple syrup

- 1/2 teaspoon ground cinnamon

- 1/4 teaspoon salt

- 1/8 teaspoon black pepper

Cooking Instructions:

- Preheat your oven to 400°F (200°C) and line a baking sheet with parchment paper.

- In a large mixing bowl, combine the butternut squash cubes, olive oil, maple syrup, cinnamon, salt, and black pepper. Toss well to evenly coat the squash with the mixture.

- Spread the butternut squash cubes in a single layer on the prepared baking sheet.

- Roast in the preheated oven for 25-30 minutes, or until the squash is fork-tender and caramelized, stirring once or twice during cooking for even browning.

- Remove the baking sheet from the oven and let the roasted butternut squash cool for a few minutes before serving.

Cooking Tips:

- Choose a ripe and firm butternut squash for best results. Look for one that is heavy for its size, with a uniform color and smooth skin.
- To make peeling and cutting the butternut squash easier, you can use a vegetable peeler to remove the skin and a sharp knife to cut it into cubes.
- Make sure to evenly coat the butternut squash with the olive oil, maple syrup, cinnamon, salt, and pepper for consistent flavor.
- You can adjust the amount of maple syrup and cinnamon to your preference. If you like it sweeter, you can add more maple syrup, or if you prefer a stronger cinnamon flavor, you can add more cinnamon.
- Be sure to keep an eye on the butternut squash while roasting to prevent burning. Cooking times may vary depending on the size and thickness of the squash cubes.
- Serve the roasted butternut squash as a side dish, or use it in salads, bowls, or as a topping for oatmeal or yogurt.

PARMESAN-ROASTED ZUCCHINI

Ingredients:

- 2 medium zucchinis, washed and sliced into 1/4-inch rounds
- 2 tablespoons olive oil
- 1/2 cup grated Parmesan cheese
- 1 teaspoon garlic powder
- 1 teaspoon dried oregano
- 1/2 teaspoon salt
- 1/4 teaspoon black pepper
- Fresh parsley, chopped (optional, for garnish)

Cooking Instructions:

- Preheat your oven to 400°F (200°C) and line a baking sheet with parchment paper.
- In a large bowl, toss the zucchini slices with olive oil, Parmesan cheese, garlic powder, dried oregano, salt, and black pepper until evenly coated.
- Arrange the coated zucchini slices in a single layer on the prepared baking sheet.
- Roast in the preheated oven for 15-20 minutes, or until the zucchini slices are tender and golden brown, flipping them halfway through to ensure even cooking.
- Remove from the oven and let cool slightly.
- Garnish with fresh chopped parsley, if desired.

- Serve the Parmesan-Roasted Zucchini as a delicious side dish or a healthy snack.

Cooking Tips:

- Use fresh zucchini for the best flavor and texture. Look for zucchinis that are firm, with smooth skin and no signs of mold or soft spots.
- You can adjust the seasonings to your preference. Add more or less Parmesan cheese, garlic powder, oregano, salt, and pepper based on your taste preferences.
- For a crispier result, you can broil the zucchini slices on high for a couple of minutes at the end of the cooking time.
- Consider using extra-virgin olive oil for its heart-healthy properties, as it contains beneficial monounsaturated fats.
- If you're watching your sodium intake, you can use a reduced-sodium or no-salt-added Parmesan cheese to lower the overall sodium content of the dish.
- Leftovers can be stored in an airtight container in the refrigerator for up to 2-3 days. To reheat, place in a preheated oven or toaster oven until warmed through and crispy.

MEDITERRANEAN COUSCOUS SALAD WITH FRESH HERBS AND FETA

Ingredients:

- 1 cup couscous
- 1 1/2 cups boiling water
- 1/2 teaspoon salt
- 1/4 teaspoon black pepper
- 1/4 cup extra-virgin olive oil
- 2 tablespoons freshly squeezed lemon juice
- 2 cloves garlic, minced
- 1/4 cup fresh parsley, chopped
- 1/4 cup fresh mint, chopped
- 1/4 cup fresh basil, chopped
- 1/2 cup cherry tomatoes, halved
- 1/2 cup cucumber, diced
- 1/4 cup red onion, finely chopped
- 1/2 cup crumbled feta cheese

Cooking Instructions:

- Place the couscous in a large heatproof bowl. Pour boiling water over the couscous, and add salt and black pepper. Stir to combine.
- Cover the bowl tightly with plastic wrap, and let the couscous stand for 5 minutes, until it has absorbed the water and is tender.
- In a small bowl, whisk together the olive oil, lemon juice, minced garlic, chopped parsley, chopped mint, and chopped basil to make the dressing.
- Fluff the cooked couscous with a fork, and then pour the dressing over the couscous. Stir gently to evenly coat the couscous with the dressing.
- Add the cherry tomatoes, cucumber, red onion, and crumbled feta cheese to the couscous. Gently stir to incorporate the ingredients.
- Taste and adjust salt and pepper as needed.
- Chill the Mediterranean couscous salad in the refrigerator for at least 30 minutes before serving to allow the flavors to meld.
- Serve the salad as a refreshing side dish or a light meal, garnished with additional herbs and feta cheese, if desired.

Cooking Tips:

- Choose whole grain couscous for added fiber and nutrients.
- If you prefer a cold salad, you can rinse the cooked couscous under cold water and let it cool completely before adding the dressing and other ingredients.
- Feel free to customize the salad by adding or substituting other Mediterranean-inspired ingredients, such as olives, roasted red peppers, artichoke hearts, or grilled vegetables.
- Use fresh herbs for the best flavor, but if fresh herbs are not available, you can use dried herbs in smaller amounts.
- To make it a complete meal, you can add cooked and cooled chickpeas or grilled chicken for added protein and fiber.
- Store leftovers in an airtight container in the refrigerator for up to 2-3 days. Stir well before serving, and add a little extra dressing if needed to refresh the flavors.

HONEY-GLAZED ROASTED CARROTS

Ingredients:

- 1 pound carrots, peeled and trimmed
- 2 tablespoons honey
- 2 tablespoons olive oil
- 1/2 teaspoon salt

- 1/4 teaspoon black pepper
- Fresh parsley, chopped (optional, for garnish)

Cooking Instructions:

- Preheat your oven to 400°F (200°C) and line a baking sheet with parchment paper for easy clean-up.
- In a large mixing bowl, whisk together the honey, olive oil, salt, and black pepper until well combined.
- Add the peeled and trimmed carrots to the bowl, and toss to coat them evenly with the honey glaze.
- Transfer the coated carrots to the prepared baking sheet, spreading them out in a single layer.
- Roast the carrots in the preheated oven for 20-25 minutes, or until they are tender and caramelized, stirring occasionally to ensure even cooking.
- Remove the carrots from the oven and let them cool for a few minutes.
- Garnish with chopped fresh parsley, if desired, before serving.

Cooking Tips:

- Choose fresh carrots that are firm and free from blemishes for the best results.

- Cut the carrots into evenly sized pieces to ensure they cook evenly.

- You can adjust the amount of honey and olive oil to your taste preferences. If you prefer a sweeter glaze, you can add more honey.

- To make this recipe vegan, you can use maple syrup or agave nectar as a substitute for honey.

- Consider using extra-virgin olive oil for its heart-healthy properties, as it contains beneficial monounsaturated fats.

- If you like, you can sprinkle some toasted sesame seeds or chopped nuts, such as almonds or pecans, over the roasted carrots for added crunch and flavor.

- Leftovers can be stored in an airtight container in the refrigerator for up to 3 days. Reheat in the oven or on the stovetop before serving.

MIXED BERRY CRISP WITH OAT TOPPING

Ingredients:

[For the Berry Filling]:

- 4 cups mixed berries (such as strawberries, blueberries, raspberries, and blackberries)
- 1/4 cup granulated sugar
- 1 tablespoon cornstarch
- 1 tablespoon freshly squeezed lemon juice

[For the Oat Topping]:

- 3/4 cup old-fashioned rolled oats
- 1/4 cup whole wheat flour
- 1/4 cup chopped nuts (such as almonds, walnuts, or pecans)
- 1/4 cup packed brown sugar
- 1/4 teaspoon ground cinnamon
- 1/4 cup cold unsalted butter, diced

Cooking Instructions:

- Preheat your oven to 350°F (175°C) and lightly grease a 9-inch square baking dish.

- In a large bowl, combine the mixed berries, granulated sugar, cornstarch, and lemon juice. Stir gently to coat the berries with the sugar mixture.

- Pour the berry mixture into the prepared baking dish and spread it out evenly.

- In a separate bowl, combine the rolled oats, whole wheat flour, chopped nuts, brown sugar, and ground cinnamon for the oat topping.

- Add the diced cold butter to the oat mixture and use a pastry cutter or your fingers to work the butter into the dry ingredients until it resembles coarse crumbs.

- Sprinkle the oat topping evenly over the berry filling in the baking dish.

- Bake the mixed berry crisp in the preheated oven for 35-40 minutes, or until the topping is golden brown and the berry filling is bubbly.

- Remove from the oven and let the crisp cool for a few minutes before serving.

- Serve warm with a scoop of low-fat vanilla yogurt or whipped cream, if desired.

Cooking Tips:

- Use a variety of mixed berries for a delicious and nutrient-rich dessert. Berries are generally low in oxalate, which is a type of mineral that can contribute to kidney stone formation, making them a good choice for kidney stone prevention.

- Adjust the amount of sugar in the recipe according to your preference and health needs. If you prefer a less sweet dessert, you can reduce the amount of sugar in the berry filling or the oat topping.

- Whole wheat flour and rolled oats provide added fiber and nutrients compared to refined flour, making them a healthier choice for the crisp topping.

- You can customize the nut selection in the oat topping based on your preference or dietary restrictions. Almonds, walnuts, and pecans are good choices for their healthy fats and crunch.

- If you're watching your fat intake, you can use a reduced-fat margarine or spread instead of butter for the oat topping, but keep in mind that the crisp may be slightly less crispy.

- Leftovers can be stored in an airtight container in the refrigerator for up to 2-3 days. Reheat before serving, if desired.

COCONUT MILK CHIA SEED PUDDING WITH FRESH FRUIT

Ingredients:

- 1/4 cup chia seeds
- 1 cup coconut milk (full-fat or light)
- 1 tablespoon pure maple syrup or honey (optional, adjust to taste)
- 1 teaspoon vanilla extract
- Fresh fruit of your choice (such as berries, mango, banana) for topping
- Unsweetened shredded coconut for garnish (optional)

Cooking Instructions:

- In a medium bowl, whisk together chia seeds, coconut milk, maple syrup or honey (if using), and vanilla extract.
- Stir well to combine, and let the mixture sit for about 5 minutes.
- Stir the chia seed mixture again to prevent clumps from forming, then cover the bowl and refrigerate for at least 4

hours or overnight, allowing the chia seeds to absorb the liquid and thicken to a pudding-like consistency.

- Once the chia seed pudding has thickened to your liking, give it a good stir.
- Serve the coconut milk chia seed pudding in individual serving bowls or glasses.
- Top with fresh fruit of your choice and garnish with shredded coconut (if using).
- Enjoy the coconut milk chia seed pudding as a nutritious and delicious dessert or breakfast option.

Cooking Tips:

- Use unsweetened coconut milk to reduce added sugars, as excessive sugar intake can contribute to kidney stone formation.
- Adjust the amount of sweetener to your preference or omit it altogether if you prefer a less sweet dessert.
- Feel free to customize the chia seed pudding with your favorite fruits, such as berries, mango, banana, or any other fresh fruits that are kidney-friendly.
- If you prefer a smoother texture, you can blend the chia seed mixture in a blender or food processor before refrigerating to create a smoother pudding consistency.

- Chia seed pudding can be stored in an airtight container in the refrigerator for up to 3-4 days. However, it's best to consume it within a day or two for optimal freshness.

GREEK YOGURT AND FRUIT PARFAIT

Ingredients:

- 1 cup plain Greek yogurt
- 1 cup mixed fresh fruits (such as berries, sliced bananas, chopped mangoes, etc.)
- 1/4 cup chopped nuts (such as almonds, walnuts, or pistachios)
- 2 tablespoons honey or pure maple syrup (optional, adjust to taste)
- 1/2 teaspoon vanilla extract
- Fresh mint leaves for garnish (optional)

Cooking Instructions:

- In a bowl or a parfait glass, layer the Greek yogurt, mixed fresh fruits, and chopped nuts.

- Repeat the layers until you use up all the ingredients or reach your desired serving size.
- Drizzle honey or pure maple syrup (if using) over the top of the parfait.
- Add a splash of vanilla extract for added flavor.
- Garnish with fresh mint leaves (if using) for a burst of freshness and visual appeal.
- Serve the Greek Yogurt and Fruit Parfait as a wholesome and kidney-friendly breakfast, snack, or dessert.

Cooking Tips:

- Use plain Greek yogurt without added sugars or flavors to reduce added sugars, as excessive sugar intake can contribute to kidney stone formation.
- Opt for mixed fresh fruits that are kidney-friendly, such as berries, bananas, mangoes, and other fruits that are low in oxalate and high in water content.
- Choose nuts that are lower in oxalate, such as almonds, walnuts, or pistachios, as some nuts, such as cashews and peanuts, are higher in oxalate and may contribute to kidney stone formation.
- Adjust the amount of sweetener to your preference or omit it altogether if you prefer a less sweet parfait.

- Feel free to customize the parfait with other kidney-friendly ingredients, such as unsweetened coconut flakes, seeds (such as chia seeds or flaxseeds), or low-oxalate fruits (such as apples or pears).

- If you have dietary restrictions or preferences, you can use a dairy-free yogurt alternative, such as coconut yogurt or almond milk yogurt, to make the parfait suitable for your needs.

- Parfaits are best consumed fresh, but you can prepare the ingredients ahead of time and assemble the parfait just before serving to maintain the desired texture and freshness.

MANGO SORBET WITH FRESH MINT

Ingredients:

- 4 ripe mangoes, peeled and chopped
- 1/2 cup water
- 1/4 cup fresh mint leaves, packed
- 1/4 cup honey or pure maple syrup (optional, adjust to taste)
- 1 tablespoon fresh lime juice

Cooking Instructions:

- In a blender or food processor, combine the chopped mangoes, water, fresh mint leaves, honey or pure maple syrup (if using), and lime juice.
- Blend or process the mixture until smooth and creamy.
- Taste and adjust the sweetness with additional honey or maple syrup if desired.
- Pour the mango sorbet mixture into an ice cream maker and churn according to the manufacturer's instructions, typically for about 20-25 minutes.
- Transfer the churned sorbet into a lidded container and freeze for at least 2-3 hours, or until firm.
- Serve the Mango Sorbet with Fresh Mint as a refreshing and kidney-friendly dessert.

Cooking Tips:

- Choose ripe mangoes for maximum natural sweetness and flavor in the sorbet. Ripe mangoes are usually slightly soft to the touch and have a fragrant aroma.
- Fresh mint leaves add a burst of freshness to the sorbet, but you can adjust the amount to your preference or omit it if you're not a fan of mint.

- If you prefer a smoother texture, you can strain the mango puree through a fine-mesh sieve to remove any fibrous bits or mint leaves.
- Adjust the amount of sweetener to your preference or omit it altogether if you prefer a less sweet sorbet. Keep in mind that excessive sugar intake can contribute to kidney stone formation, so it's important to monitor your added sugar intake.
- You can also use a natural sugar substitute, such as stevia or erythritol, as a sweetener alternative if you have dietary restrictions or preferences.
- Enjoy the Mango Sorbet with Fresh Mint in moderation as a treat, and remember to stay hydrated and follow a kidney-friendly diet as recommended by your healthcare provider or a registered dietitian for kidney stone prevention.

BERRY AND GREEK YOGURT SMOOTHIE

Ingredients:

- 1 cup mixed berries (such as strawberries, blueberries, raspberries, or blackberries)
- 1 cup plain Greek yogurt

- 1/2 cup water or unsweetened almond milk
- 1 tablespoon honey or pure maple syrup (optional, adjust to taste)
- 1/2 teaspoon vanilla extract
- Ice cubes (optional)

Cooking Instructions:

- Wash the berries thoroughly and remove any stems or leaves.
- In a blender, add the mixed berries, Greek yogurt, water or almond milk, honey or pure maple syrup (if using), and vanilla extract.
- If desired, add a few ice cubes to chill the smoothie and make it frosty.
- Blend on high speed until smooth and creamy.
- Taste and adjust the sweetness with more honey or maple syrup, if desired.
- Pour the Berry and Greek Yogurt Smoothie into glasses and serve immediately.

Cooking Tips:

- Use plain Greek yogurt without added sugars or flavors to reduce added sugars, as excessive sugar intake can contribute to kidney stone formation.

- Opt for mixed berries that are kidney-friendly, such as strawberries, blueberries, raspberries, or blackberries, as they are low in oxalate and high in antioxidants and vitamins.

- Adjust the amount of sweetener to your preference or omit it altogether if you prefer a less sweet smoothie.

- You can use water or unsweetened almond milk as the liquid base for the smoothie. Avoid using high-oxalate liquids like beet juice or spinach juice, as they may increase the oxalate content of the smoothie.

- If you have dietary restrictions or preferences, you can use a dairy-free yogurt alternative, such as coconut yogurt or almond milk yogurt, to make the smoothie suitable for your needs.

- Feel free to customize the smoothie with other kidney-friendly ingredients, such as spinach, kale, or seeds (such as chia seeds or flaxseeds), for added nutrition.

- Smoothies are best consumed fresh, but you can prepare the ingredients ahead of time and blend the smoothie just before serving to maintain the desired texture and freshness.

DARK CHOCOLATE AND ALMOND BARK

Ingredients:

- 8 oz dark chocolate (70% cocoa or higher), chopped
- 1 cup raw almonds, roughly chopped
- 1/4 teaspoon sea salt (optional)
- 1 tablespoon pure maple syrup or honey (optional)

Cooking Instructions:

- Line a baking sheet or a rectangular baking dish with parchment paper.
- In a heatproof bowl, melt the dark chocolate over a double boiler or in short intervals in the microwave, stirring frequently to avoid burning.
- Once the chocolate is fully melted and smooth, remove from heat and stir in the chopped almonds.
- Pour the chocolate and almond mixture onto the prepared baking sheet or dish, spreading it evenly with a spatula.
- Sprinkle sea salt (if using) evenly over the top for a touch of savory contrast (optional).

- Drizzle pure maple syrup or honey (if using) over the top for added sweetness (optional).
- Place the baking sheet or dish in the refrigerator for at least 30 minutes, or until the chocolate is fully set.
- Once set, break the dark chocolate and almond bark into desired pieces or shards.
- Store the bark in an airtight container in the refrigerator until ready to serve.

Cooking Tips:

- Choose dark chocolate with a cocoa content of 70% or higher, as it contains less sugar and higher levels of antioxidants compared to milk or white chocolate.
- Use raw almonds for their natural crunch and nutritional benefits. You can also use other nuts, such as walnuts or pecans, if desired.
- Consider adding a touch of sea salt for a savory contrast to the sweetness of the dark chocolate, but be mindful of your sodium intake if you have kidney stone issues or other health conditions.
- You can drizzle a small amount of pure maple syrup or honey over the top of the bark for added sweetness, but use

it sparingly as excessive sugar intake may contribute to kidney stone formation.

- Enjoy the dark chocolate and almond bark in moderation as a kidney-friendly treat, as excessive consumption of dark chocolate or almonds may not be suitable for everyone, especially those with specific dietary restrictions or health conditions.

- Feel free to customize the bark with other kidney-friendly ingredients, such as dried fruits (such as apricots or raisins), seeds (such as chia seeds or flaxseeds), or other nuts/seeds with lower oxalate content, depending on your specific dietary needs or preferences.

FRUIT SALAD WITH HONEY-LIME DRESSING

Ingredients:

- Assorted fresh fruits (such as berries, melons, citrus fruits, grapes, etc.), washed and chopped
- 2 tablespoons fresh lime juice
- 2 tablespoons raw honey
- 1/2 teaspoon finely grated lime zest
- Fresh mint leaves, for garnish (optional)

Cooking Instructions:

- Wash and chop a variety of fresh fruits of your choice, such as berries, melons, citrus fruits, grapes, etc. and place them in a large serving bowl.
- In a small bowl, whisk together fresh lime juice, raw honey, and finely grated lime zest to make the dressing.
- Drizzle the honey-lime dressing over the chopped fruits in the serving bowl.
- Gently toss the fruits with the dressing until well coated.
- Garnish the fruit salad with fresh mint leaves, if desired.
- Serve the fruit salad immediately and enjoy!

Cooking Tips:

- Choose a variety of fresh fruits with lower oxalate content, such as berries, melons, and citrus fruits, as they may be more kidney-friendly compared to fruits with higher oxalate levels, such as bananas, strawberries, or kiwis.
- Be mindful of portion sizes and moderation, as excessive consumption of fruits, even those with lower oxalate content, may not be suitable for everyone, especially those with specific dietary restrictions or health conditions.

- Use raw honey or other natural sweeteners instead of refined sugars to control sugar intake and avoid excessive sugar consumption, which may contribute to kidney stone formation.
- Fresh lime juice and zest add a tangy flavor to the dressing, but you can also use lemon juice and zest as a substitute.
- Consider adding fresh mint leaves for a refreshing and aromatic twist, but be mindful of your sodium intake if you have kidney stone issues or other health conditions.
- Feel free to customize the fruit salad with other kidney-friendly ingredients, such as seeds (such as chia seeds or flaxseeds), nuts (such as almonds or walnuts), or other fruits with lower oxalate content, depending on your specific dietary needs or preferences.
- Always consult with your healthcare provider or a registered dietitian for personalized dietary recommendations based on your specific health needs, including kidney stone prevention.

COCONUT WATER WITH FRESH LIME AND MINT

Ingredients:

- 1 cup coconut water
- Juice of 1 fresh lime
- 1 tablespoon freshly chopped mint leaves
- Ice cubes (optional)

Cooking Instructions:

- In a glass, combine coconut water, fresh lime juice, and freshly chopped mint leaves.
- Stir well to combine the ingredients.
- Add ice cubes, if desired, to chill the drink.
- Garnish with a sprig of mint leaves for presentation (optional).
- Enjoy the refreshing and hydrating Coconut Water with Fresh Lime and Mint!

Cooking Tips:

- Choose pure coconut water without added sugars or flavors for a healthier option. Look for brands that use minimal processing and do not contain added preservatives or artificial ingredients.

- Freshly squeezed lime juice is recommended for maximum flavor and health benefits. You can adjust the amount of lime juice to suit your taste preferences.
- Fresh mint leaves add a refreshing and aromatic twist to the drink. You can adjust the amount of mint leaves based on your preference for the mint flavor.
- You can also muddle the mint leaves with a muddler or the back of a spoon to release more of the mint's flavor before adding it to the coconut water and lime juice.
- Consider using chilled coconut water and freshly squeezed lime juice for a colder and more refreshing drink. You can also chill the glass and coconut water in the refrigerator beforehand for an extra cold drink.
- If you prefer a sweeter taste, you can add a small amount of raw honey or other natural sweeteners to the drink, but be mindful of your sugar intake, especially if you have kidney stone issues or other health conditions.

PINEAPPLE AND COCONUT MILK SMOOTHIE

Ingredients:

- 1 cup frozen pineapple chunks

- 1 cup unsweetened coconut milk
- 1 tablespoon raw honey (optional)
- 1/2 teaspoon grated fresh ginger (optional)
- 1/2 cup ice cubes

Cooking Instructions:

- Add frozen pineapple chunks, unsweetened coconut milk, raw honey (if using), grated fresh ginger (if using), and ice cubes to a blender.
- Blend on high speed until the mixture is smooth and creamy.
- Taste and adjust sweetness with additional honey, if desired.
- Pour the smoothie into glasses and serve immediately.

Cooking Tips:

- Use frozen pineapple chunks to create a thick and creamy smoothie. You can also use fresh pineapple, but the smoothie may be thinner in consistency.
- Choose unsweetened coconut milk to control sugar intake and avoid excessive sugar consumption, which may contribute to kidney stone formation.

- You can add raw honey or other natural sweeteners to taste, but be mindful of your sugar intake and consult with your healthcare provider or a registered dietitian for personalized dietary recommendations based on your specific health needs.
- Fresh ginger adds a tangy and spicy flavor to the smoothie and may have potential health benefits, including anti-inflammatory properties. However, if you have kidney stone issues or other health conditions, consult with your healthcare provider before adding ginger to your diet.
- Consider adding some greens, such as baby spinach or kale, to the smoothie for an extra nutrient boost. However, be mindful of oxalate content in greens and choose those with lower oxalate levels if you have kidney stone issues.

GREEK YOGURT AND BERRY FROZEN POPSICLES

Ingredients:

- 1 cup plain Greek yogurt
- 1 cup mixed berries (such as blueberries, strawberries, raspberries, or blackberries), washed and hulled
- 2 tablespoons raw honey or other natural sweeteners

- 1/2 teaspoon pure vanilla extract (optional)
- Popsicle molds
- Popsicle sticks

Cooking Instructions:

- In a blender or food processor, combine Greek yogurt, mixed berries, raw honey or other natural sweeteners, and pure vanilla extract (if using).
- Blend the mixture until smooth and well combined.
- Taste the mixture and adjust the sweetness level with additional honey or sweeteners, if desired.
- Pour the yogurt and berry mixture into popsicle molds, leaving a small gap at the top to allow for expansion during freezing.
- Insert popsicle sticks into the molds.
- Place the popsicle molds in the freezer and freeze for at least 4-6 hours or until fully frozen.
- Once frozen, carefully remove the popsicles from the molds by running them under warm water for a few seconds to loosen them, then gently pull them out.
- Serve the Greek Yogurt and Berry Frozen Popsicles immediately and enjoy!

Cooking Tips:

- Choose plain Greek yogurt with low or no added sugars to control sugar intake and avoid excessive sugar consumption, which may contribute to kidney stone formation.

- Use a variety of mixed berries with lower oxalate content, such as blueberries, strawberries, raspberries, or blackberries, as they may be more kidney-friendly compared to fruits with higher oxalate levels, such as bananas, kiwis, or figs.

- Adjust the sweetness level of the popsicles to your liking by using raw honey or other natural sweeteners, and taste the mixture before freezing to ensure it meets your preferences.

- Add pure vanilla extract for additional flavor, if desired, but be mindful of your sodium intake if you have kidney stone issues or other health conditions.

- If you don't have popsicle molds, you can also use small paper cups or ice cube trays as alternatives. Just insert popsicle sticks or small wooden sticks into the cups or trays before freezing.

- Consider adding other kidney-friendly ingredients, such as nuts (such as almonds or walnuts) or seeds (such as chia seeds or flaxseeds), to the popsicles for added texture and nutrition, depending on your specific dietary needs or preferences.

CHAPTER 5: MEAL PLAN, SHOPPING LISTS, AND FOOD LABEL READING

28-Day Meal Plan

Day 1:

Morning: Blueberry Spinach Smoothie

Lunch: Lentil and Vegetable Soup

Dinner: Veggie Burger with Sweet Potato Fries

Snack/Dessert: Greek Yogurt and Fruit Parfait

Day 2:

Morning: Veggie Omelette with Spinach and Mushrooms

Lunch: Greek Salad with Grilled Chicken and Lemon Dressing

Dinner: Tofu and Vegetable Curry with Brown Rice

Snack/Dessert: Mixed Berry Crisp with Oat Topping

Day 3:

Morning: Quinoa Breakfast Bowl with Fresh Fruit

Lunch: Kale Caesar Salad with Grilled Salmon

Dinner: Baked Cod with Herbs and Tomatoes

Snack/Dessert: Coconut Milk Chia Seed Pudding with Fresh Fruit

Day 4:

Morning: Greek Yogurt Parfait with Berries and Nuts

Lunch: Quinoa and Veggie Salad with Lemon-Herb Dressing

Dinner: Lentil and Vegetable Stir-Fry with Ginger and Soy Sauce

Snack/Dessert: Mango Sorbet with Fresh Mint

Day 5:

Morning: Avocado and Egg Toast

Lunch: Sweet Potato and Black Bean Salad with Lime Vinaigrette

Dinner: Grilled Portobello Mushrooms with Balsamic Glaze

Snack/Dessert: Berry and Greek Yogurt Smoothie

Day 6:

Morning: Berry Chia Seed Pudding

Lunch: Gazpacho with Fresh Tomatoes and Cucumbers

Dinner: Lemon-Rosemary Roasted Turkey Breast with Roasted Vegetables

Snack/Dessert: Dark Chocolate and Almond Bark

Day 7:

Morning: Sweet Potato Hash with Kale and Eggs

Lunch: Thai Chicken Salad with Peanut Dressing

Dinner: Spaghetti Squash with Tomato Sauce and Turkey Meatballs

Snack/Dessert: Fruit Salad with Honey-Lime Dressing

Day 8:

Morning: Green Smoothie Bowl with Kale, Banana, and Almond Milk

Lunch: Minestrone Soup with Vegetables and Beans

Dinner: Teriyaki Chicken with Steamed Vegetables and Brown Rice

Snack/Dessert: Greek Yogurt and Berry Frozen Popsicles

Day 9:

Morning: Buckwheat Pancakes with Fresh Berries

Lunch: Lentil and Vegetable Soup

Dinner: Black Bean and Sweet Potato Enchiladas with Avocado Cream Sauce

Snack/Dessert: Coconut Water with Fresh Lime and Mint

Day 10:

Morning: Spinach and Mushroom Frittata

Lunch: Greek Salad with Grilled Chicken and Lemon Dressing

Dinner: Veggie Burger with Sweet Potato Fries

Snack/Dessert: Mixed Berry Crisp with Oat Topping

Morning: Breakfast Burrito with Black Beans, Avocado, and Salsa

Lunch: Quinoa and Veggie Salad with Lemon-Herb Dressing

Dinner: Baked Cod with Herbs and Tomatoes

Snack/Dessert: Greek Yogurt and Fruit Parfait

Morning: Oatmeal with Fresh Fruit and Almonds

Lunch: Sweet Potato and Black Bean Salad with Lime Vinaigrette

Dinner: Tofu and Vegetable Curry with Brown Rice

Snack/Dessert: Mango Sorbet with Fresh Mint

Morning: Coconut Milk and Mango Smoothie

Lunch: Kale Caesar Salad with Grilled Salmon

Dinner: Lentil and Vegetable Stir-Fry with Ginger and Soy Sauce

Day 14:

Breakfast: Berry Chia Seed Pudding

Snack: Fresh Fruit Salad with Mint and Lime

Lunch: Lentil and Vegetable Soup

Snack: Greek Yogurt and Fruit Parfait

Dinner: Baked Cod with Herbs and Tomatoes, served with Steamed Broccoli with Garlic and Olive Oil

Dessert: Fruit Salad with Honey-Lime Dressing

Day 15:

Breakfast: Greek Yogurt Parfait with Berries and Nuts

Snack: Edamame with Sea Salt

Lunch: Butternut Squash Soup with Coconut Milk and Ginger, served with Mediterranean Couscous Salad with Fresh Herbs and Feta

Snack: Pineapple and Coconut Milk Smoothie

Dinner: Veggie Burger with Sweet Potato Fries

Dessert: Mixed Berry Crisp with Oat Topping

Breakfast: Quinoa Breakfast Bowl with Fresh Fruit

Snack: Roasted Chickpeas with Herbs and Spices

Lunch: Thai Chicken Salad with Peanut Dressing

Snack: Greek Yogurt and Berry Frozen Popsicles

Dinner: Greek-style Grilled Lamb Chops with Mediterranean Couscous and Roasted Cauliflower

Dessert: Mango Sorbet with Fresh Mint

Breakfast: Veggie Omelette with Spinach and Mushrooms

Snack: Caprese Salad with Tomatoes, Fresh Mozzarella, and Basil

Lunch: Lentil and Vegetable Stir-Fry with Ginger and Soy Sauce, served with Cilantro-Lime Brown Rice

Snack: Dark Chocolate and Almond Bark

Dinner: Lemon-Rosemary Roasted Turkey Breast with Roasted Vegetables

Dessert: Coconut Milk Chia Seed Pudding with Fresh Fruit

Day 18:

Breakfast: Avocado and Egg Toast

Snack: Avocado and Tomato Bruschetta

Lunch: Tuna Salad with Mixed Greens and Lemon-Dijon Dressing

Snack: Greek Hummus with Fresh Vegetables

Dinner: Spaghetti Squash with Tomato Sauce and Turkey Meatballs, served with Garlic-Sauteed Spinach

Dessert: Greek Yogurt and Fruit Parfait

Day 19:

Breakfast: Green Smoothie Bowl with Kale, Banana, and Almond Milk

Snack: Sweet Potato Chips with Rosemary and Sea Salt

Lunch: Greek Salad with Grilled Chicken and Lemon Dressing

Snack: Coconut Water with Fresh Lime and Mint

Dinner: Black Bean and Sweet Potato Enchiladas with Avocado Cream Sauce

Dessert: Fruit Salad with Honey-Lime Dressing

Day 20:

Breakfast: Buckwheat Pancakes with Fresh Berries

Snack: Veggie Sushi Rolls with Brown Rice and Avocado

Lunch: Quinoa and Veggie Salad with Lemon-Herb Dressing

Snack: Greek Yogurt and Berry Smoothie

Dinner: Tofu and Vegetable Curry with Brown Rice

Dessert: Mixed Berry Crisp with Oat Topping

Day 21:

Breakfast: Spinach and Mushroom Frittata

Snack: Sweet Potato Chips with Rosemary and Sea Salt

Lunch: Gazpacho with Fresh Tomatoes and Cucumbers, served with Beet and Goat Cheese Salad with Walnuts and Balsamic Glaze

Snack: Fruit Salad with Honey-Lime Dressing

Dinner: Grilled Portobello Mushrooms with Balsamic Glaze, served with Parmesan-Roasted Zucchini

Dessert: Coconut Milk Chia Seed Pudding with Fresh Fruit

Day 22:

Breakfast: Breakfast Burrito with Black Beans, Avocado, and Salsa

Snack: Greek Yogurt with Honey and Mixed Nuts

Lunch: Lentil and Vegetable Stir-Fry with Ginger and Soy Sauce, served with Quinoa

Snack: Fresh Fruit Smoothie with Spinach and Banana

Dinner: Grilled Salmon with Lemon-Dill Sauce, served with Roasted Brussels Sprouts with Balsamic Glaze and Quinoa

Dessert: Dark Chocolate and Mixed Berry Parfait with Greek Yogurt

Day 23:

Breakfast: Overnight Oats with Berries and Almonds

Snack: Roasted Chickpeas with Herbs and Spices

Lunch: Mediterranean Veggie Wrap with Hummus and Feta Cheese

Snack: Fresh Fruit Salad with Mint and Lime

Dinner: Stuffed Bell Peppers with Quinoa, Black Beans, and Veggies, served with Cilantro-Lime Brown Rice

Dessert: Mixed Berry Smoothie with Greek Yogurt and Honey

Day 24:

Breakfast: Veggie Omelette with Spinach, Tomatoes, and Cheese

Snack: Greek Yogurt with Fresh Fruit and Granola

Lunch: Thai Coconut Curry with Vegetables and Tofu, served with Jasmine Rice

Snack: Roasted Edamame with Sea Salt

Dinner: Grilled Chicken Breast with Lemon-Rosemary Marinade, served with Garlic-Roasted Asparagus and Quinoa

Dessert: Mango Sorbet with Fresh Mint

Day 25:

Breakfast: Banana and Almond Butter Smoothie with Spinach

Snack: Greek Yogurt and Berry Frozen Popsicles

Lunch: Lentil and Vegetable Soup with Whole Grain Bread

Snack: Fresh Fruit Salad with Honey-Lime Dressing

Dinner: Quinoa and Veggie Stir-Fry with Teriyaki Sauce

Dessert: Coconut Milk Chia Seed Pudding with Fresh Fruit

Day 26:

Breakfast: Avocado and Egg Toast with Tomatoes and Sprouts

Snack: Mixed Nuts and Dried Fruit Trail Mix

Lunch: Mediterranean Chickpea Salad with Tomatoes, Cucumbers, and Feta Cheese, served with Whole Grain Pita Bread

Snack: Greek Yogurt with Honey and Mixed Berries

Dinner: Grilled Veggie Skewers with Balsamic Glaze, served with Lemon-Parsley Couscous

Dessert: Dark Chocolate and Almond Bark

Day 27:

Breakfast: Berry Protein Smoothie with Greek Yogurt and Spinach

Snack: Caprese Salad with Tomatoes, Fresh Mozzarella, and Basil

Lunch: Lentil and Vegetable Curry with Coconut Milk, served with Brown Rice

Snack: Fresh Fruit Salad with Mint and Lime

Dinner: Baked Cod with Lemon-Dill Sauce, served with Roasted Vegetables and Quinoa

Dessert: Greek Yogurt Parfait with Berries and Nuts

Day 28:

Breakfast: Green Smoothie Bowl with Kale, Banana, and Almond Milk

Snack: Sweet Potato Chips with Rosemary and Sea Salt

Lunch: Quinoa and Veggie Salad with Lemon-Herb Dressing

Snack: Greek Yogurt with Fresh Fruit and Granola

Dinner: Veggie Burger with Sweet Potato Fries

Dessert: Mixed Berry Crisp with Oat Topping

This a great sample meal plan to help you get started on your dieting journey against Kidney Stones. It doesn't have to stop here though.

If you feel the need to, or you have other medical complications, consulting for the advice of a registered dietitian near you would be highly recommended by me. That way, a more personalized meal plan can be set up to tailor your medical and health needs.

Shopping Lists for Kidney Stone Diet

Maintaining a kidney stone diet requires careful planning and grocery shopping to ensure that you are consuming foods that are kidney stone friendly and avoiding those that are not. Here are some detailed shopping lists that you can use as a reference when you head to the grocery store to stock up on kidney stone friendly foods.

Fresh Produce:

Leafy greens such as spinach, kale, and Swiss chard: These are excellent sources of calcium, which can help bind oxalate in the gut and prevent it from being absorbed into the bloodstream, reducing the risk of oxalate-based kidney stone formation.

Citrus fruits such as oranges, lemons, and limes: These are rich in citrate, which can inhibit the formation of calcium-based kidney stones.

Berries such as strawberries, blueberries, and raspberries: These are low in oxalate and high in fiber, making them healthy choices for a kidney stone diet.

Cruciferous vegetables such as broccoli, cauliflower, and cabbage: These are low in oxalate and packed with nutrients, making them great options for a kidney stone friendly diet.

Low-Oxalate Grains:

Brown rice: This is a low-oxalate grain that can be used as a base for many meals, such as stir-fries, salads, and grain bowls.

Quinoa: This is another low-oxalate grain that is high in protein and fiber, making it a healthy addition to a kidney stone friendly diet.

Whole grain bread: Look for bread that is made with whole grains, such as wheat, oats, or rye, and does not contain added nuts or seeds, which can be high in oxalate.

Lean Proteins:

Chicken breast: This is a lean source of protein that can be grilled, roasted, or sautéed for a variety of kidney stone friendly meals.

Fish: Look for low-oxalate fish options such as salmon, trout, and tilapia, which are also excellent sources of omega-3 fatty acids.

Eggs: Eggs are a great source of protein and can be used in many kidney stone friendly recipes, such as omelets, frittatas, and egg salads.

Tofu: This is a plant-based source of protein that is low in oxalate and can be used in a variety of kidney stone friendly dishes, such as stir-fries, curries, and salads.

Dairy and Dairy Alternatives:

Low-fat or fat-free milk: Milk is a good source of calcium and can be used in moderation as part of a kidney stone diet. Opt for low-fat or fat-free options to reduce saturated fat intake.

Greek yogurt: This is a good source of protein and calcium, but be sure to choose plain or low-sugar varieties to avoid added sugars.

Cheese: Look for low-fat or reduced-fat cheese options, such as mozzarella, ricotta, and feta, which are lower in oxalate compared to other types of cheese.

Dairy alternatives: If you are lactose intolerant or prefer dairy alternatives, choose options such as almond milk, coconut milk, or rice milk that are fortified with calcium.

Water: Staying well-hydrated is important for kidney stone prevention, so make sure to drink plenty of water throughout the day. Keep a reusable water bottle with you to stay hydrated on the go.

Herbal teas: Some herbal teas, such as nettle leaf tea, have been shown to have potential benefits in reducing the risk of kidney stone formation. Choose caffeine-free options and avoid teas that contain ingredients high in oxalate, such as black tea or green tea.

Lemon or lime juice: Adding a splash of lemon or lime juice to your water or herbal tea can help increase citrate levels in the urine, which can help prevent kidney stone formation.

Low-sugar fruit juices: Look for fruit juices that are low in added sugars and are made from kidney stone friendly fruits such as citrus fruits, berries, and melons.

Nuts and seeds: Choose low-oxalate options such as almonds, sunflower seeds, and flaxseeds for a healthy and kidney stone friendly snack option.

Hummus: Made from chickpeas, which are low in oxalate, hummus can be a delicious and nutritious dip for vegetables or whole grain crackers.

Nut butters: Opt for nut butters made from low-oxalate nuts such as almond or sunflower seed butter, and enjoy them in moderation as a spread or dip.

Fresh herbs and spices: Herbs and spices can add flavor to your meals without adding oxalate or sodium. Choose fresh options such as basil, thyme, oregano, and ginger for a kidney stone friendly diet.

Vinegar: Vinegar, such as apple cider vinegar or balsamic vinegar, can be used in moderation as a low-oxalate dressing for salads or marinades.

Other Kidney Stone Friendly Foods:

Legumes: Beans, lentils, and peas are low in oxalate and high in fiber and protein, making them excellent choices for a kidney stone diet.

Avocado: This creamy fruit is low in oxalate and high in healthy fats, making it a nutritious option for a kidney stone friendly diet.

Coconut oil: Coconut oil is a healthy fat that can be used for cooking and baking, and it is low in oxalate.

Dark chocolate: Look for dark chocolate with low sugar content and enjoy it in moderation as a kidney stone friendly treat.

Foods to Limit or Avoid:

High-oxalate foods: Foods that are high in oxalate, such as spinach, beets, sweet potatoes, and nuts like almonds and cashews, should be consumed in moderation or avoided in a kidney stone diet.

Processed foods: Processed foods, such as packaged snacks, fast food, and processed meats, tend to be high in sodium, unhealthy fats, and added sugars, which can increase the risk of kidney stone formation.

Sugary beverages: Beverages that are high in added sugars, such as soda, energy drinks, and fruit juices with added sugars, should be limited or avoided in a kidney stone diet.

High-sodium foods: Foods that are high in sodium, such as canned soups, processed meats, and salty snacks, can increase the risk of kidney stone formation. Choose low-sodium options whenever possible.

Food Label Reading for Kidney Stone Diet

When following a kidney stone diet, it's important to pay attention to the nutritional content of the foods you consume. One effective way to do this is by reading and understanding food labels. Food labels provide valuable information about the nutrients and ingredients in a product, helping you make informed choices that align with your kidney stone friendly diet. Here are some tips on how to read food labels effectively:

Check the Serving Size: The serving size listed on the food label is the amount of the product that the nutrition information is based on. It's important to pay attention to the serving size, as it determines the amount of nutrients and oxalate you'll be consuming. Be mindful of portion sizes and consider how much you typically consume in one sitting.

Look for Oxalate Content: One of the key nutrients to monitor in a kidney stone diet is oxalate. Oxalate is found in many foods and can contribute to the formation of kidney stones in susceptible individuals. Look for the oxalate content listed on the food label, and choose foods that are low in oxalate or fit within your recommended oxalate intake as advised by your healthcare provider or registered dietitian.

Pay Attention to Sodium Content: Sodium is another nutrient to watch out for in a kidney stone diet, as it can increase the risk of kidney stone formation. Look for the sodium content on the food label, and choose foods that are low in sodium or fit within your recommended sodium intake as advised by your healthcare provider or registered dietitian.

Check Total and Added Sugars: Sugar intake should also be monitored in a kidney stone diet, as excessive sugar consumption can lead to weight gain and other health issues. Look for the total and added sugars listed on the food label. Choose foods that are low in total and added sugars, and opt for natural sugar sources such as fruits over added sugars like high-fructose corn syrup.

Assess Fat Content: While healthy fats are important for overall health, it's still essential to monitor your fat intake, especially if you have a history of kidney stones. Look for the total fat content on the food label and choose foods that are low in unhealthy fats such as saturated and trans fats. Opt for healthy fats such as monounsaturated and polyunsaturated fats found in nuts, seeds, avocados, and fatty fish.

Consider Fiber and Protein: Fiber and protein are important nutrients for a healthy kidney stone diet. Look for foods that are rich in fiber and protein, such as whole grains, legumes, nuts, seeds, and lean meats or plant-based protein sources. These nutrients can help you feel fuller for longer and support healthy digestion.

Read Ingredient List: The ingredient list on a food label provides valuable information about the components of a product. Avoid foods that contain high-oxalate ingredients such as spinach, beets, and nuts if you are trying to reduce your oxalate intake. Also, be cautious of foods with added sugars, sodium, and unhealthy fats in the ingredient list.

Watch for Hidden Sodium: Sodium can sometimes be hidden in processed foods under various names, such as monosodium glutamate (MSG), sodium bicarbonate, sodium nitrite, and sodium benzoate. Be vigilant and look for these hidden sources of sodium in the ingredient list.

Consider Food Additives: Some food additives, such as citric acid and ascorbic acid, can increase the citrate levels in urine, which may help prevent kidney stone formation. Look for foods that contain kidney stone friendly additives, but be cautious of other additives that may be harmful to your overall health.

Seek Professional Advice: If you're unsure about certain foods or how to interpret food labels, it's always best to consult with a registered dietitian or healthcare provider who can provide personalized guidance based on your specific kidney stone diet needs.

In conclusion, understanding how to read food labels is a valuable skill for anyone following a kidney stone diet. By checking the serving size, oxalate content, sodium content, sugars, fats, fiber, protein, ingredient list, hidden sodium, and food additives, you can make informed choices about the foods you consume and ensure they align with your kidney stone friendly diet goals.

Always remember to seek professional advice if you have any questions or concerns about specific foods or food labels. With careful attention to food labels, you can make smart choices and support your kidney stone diet journey. Happy label reading!

CHAPTER 6: CONCLUSION AND RESOURCES

Congratulations! You've reached the end of the KIDNEY STONE DIET COOKBOOK. By now, you have gained a comprehensive understanding of kidney stones and how dietary modifications can play a crucial role in preventing and reversing their formation. I hope that this cookbook has been a valuable resource in guiding you towards a healthy, kidney-friendly diet that can help you prevent kidney stones and support your overall kidney health.

Throughout this cookbook, I have covered a wide range of topics, including the types of kidney stones, their causes, risk factors, and symptoms. I have also provided detailed information about various nutrients, minerals, and dietary factors that can impact kidney stone formation. With this knowledge, you are now empowered to make informed choices when it comes to planning your meals and making dietary changes.

I have also shared numerous delicious and nutritious recipes that are specifically designed to support kidney health and reduce the risk of kidney stone formation. From scrumptious breakfast options to satisfying main courses, and delightful desserts, these recipes showcase a wide variety of flavorful ingredients that are beneficial for your kidneys. I have emphasized the importance of hydration, portion control, and moderation in your dietary choices, and provided tips on how to incorporate kidney-friendly foods into your daily routine.

It is important to remember that reversing and preventing kidney stones is a lifelong commitment. By following the dietary recommendations provided in this cookbook, along with adopting other healthy lifestyle habits, such as regular physical activity, managing stress, and avoiding tobacco and excessive alcohol consumption, you can take proactive steps to promote kidney health and reduce the risk of kidney stone formation.

In addition to dietary modifications, I also encourage you to work closely with your healthcare provider, including a registered dietitian or nutritionist, to develop a personalized kidney stone prevention/treatment plan that is tailored to your individual needs and medical history. They can provide you with expert advice, monitor your progress, and make necessary adjustments to your diet to ensure optimal kidney health.

By making the right dietary choices and taking steps to protect your kidneys, you are investing in your long-term health and well-being. I sincerely hope that this book, the KIDNEY STONE DIET

COOKBOOK has been a valuable tool in your journey towards better kidney health, and that you continue to prioritize your kidneys by making healthy dietary choices every day.

Thank you for joining me on this culinary adventure, and here's to a future of healthy kidneys and a vibrant, fulfilling life! Bon appétit!

IF YOU HAVE BENEFITTED FROM THIS BOOK, KINDLY GIVE ME A NICE REVIEW ON AMAZON. IT WILL HELP MORE KIDNEY STONES PATIENTS SEE MY DIET SOLUTIONS PROVIDED IN THIS BOOK EASILY.

OTHER OF MY KIDNEY HEALTH BOOKS ON AMAZON YOU MIGHT BE INTERESTED IN INCLUDE:

See next page ➡

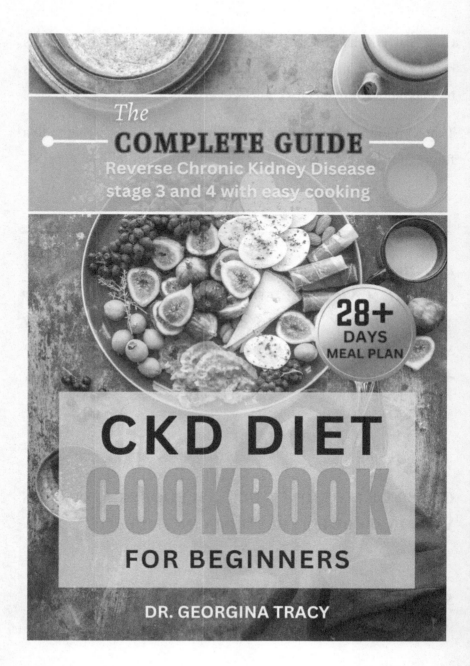

The
COMPLETE GUIDE
Reverse Chronic Kidney Disease
stage 3 and 4 with easy cooking

28+
DAYS
MEAL PLAN

CKD DIET
COOKBOOK
FOR BEGINNERS

DR. GEORGINA TRACY

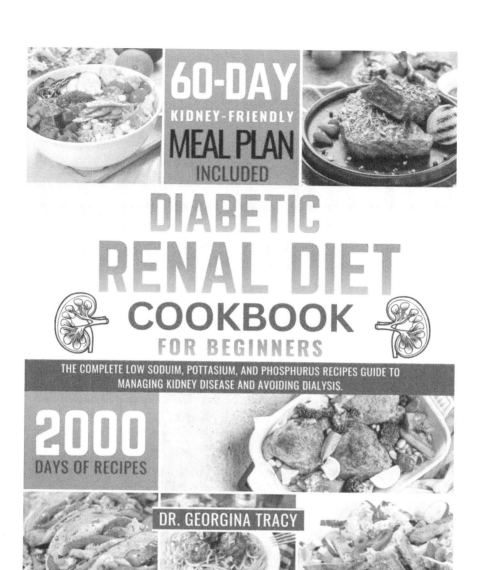

60-DAY
KIDNEY-FRIENDLY
MEAL PLAN
INCLUDED

DIABETIC
RENAL DIET
COOKBOOK
FOR BEGINNERS

THE COMPLETE LOW SODUIM, POTTASIUM, AND PHOSPHURUS RECIPES GUIDE TO
MANAGING KIDNEY DISEASE AND AVOIDING DIALYSIS.

2000
DAYS OF RECIPES

DR. GEORGINA TRACY

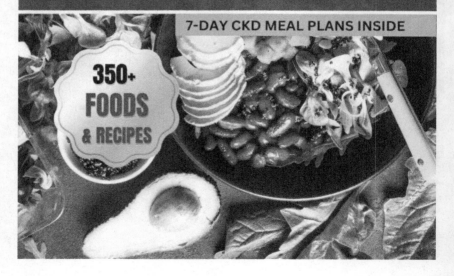

ABOUT THE AUTHOR

Dr. Georgina Tracy is a Registered Dietitian Nutritionist and researcher specializing in chronic illnesses including cancer, CKD, and hepatitis. She has a Master's degree in Biochemistry and a PhD in Nutrition, and has worked in both private and public practice, research, and teaching for over 25 years. Her research experience includes studies on dietary intake, nutrient metabolism, and disease prevention - as well as reversal.

Dr. Georgina is dedicated to providing evidence-based nutrition care that is both effective and accessible to everyone. She is passionate about helping individuals reach their health goals and living their best life. Her books are an easy-to-use guide to help you make the most of your nutrition and lifestyle choices.

Made in the USA
Las Vegas, NV
06 December 2023

82211033R00144